**Oral Health in Germany:
Diagnostic Criteria and Data Recording Manual**
Materialienreihe
Band 11.2

J. Einwag/K. Keß/E. Reich

Oral Health in Germany: Diagnostic Criteria and Data Recording Manual

Instructions for examination and documentation of oral health status

– With an appendix of the sociological survey instruments for the assessment of oral health attitudes and behaviour –

Foreword by R. Naujoks

edited by:
Institut der Deutschen Zahnärzte
under the aegis of
Bundesverband der Deutschen Zahnärztekammern e.V. – Bundeszahnärztekammer
(German Dental Association)
Kassenzahnärztliche Bundesvereinigung K.d.ö.R
(Panel Dentists' Federal Association)
D 5000 Köln 41, Universitätsstraße 71–73

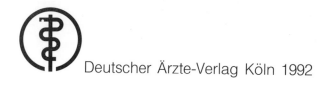

Deutscher Ärzte-Verlag Köln 1992

Institut der Deutschen Zahnärzte in collaboration with the dental experts associated with the research project

"Representative population survey of oral health status and oral hygiene practice in the Federal Republic of Germany"

Authors of the Manual:

Priv.-Doz. Dr. Johannes Einwag
Department of Restorative Dentistry and Periodontology
University of Würzburg

Dr. Klaus Keß
Department of Orthodontics
University of Würzburg

Dr. Elmar Reich
Department of Restorative Dentistry and Periodontology
University of Regensburg

Foreword:

Prof. Dr. Rudolf Naujoks
former Director of the School of Dental Medicine
University of Würzburg

English Translation:

Philip Slotkin M.A. Cantab M.I.T.I.
London

Editorial Work:

Dorothee Fink
Institute of German Dentists
Cologne

ISBN 3-7691-7826-2

All rights reserved. No part of this publication may be reproduced, stored in a retrieval system, or transmitted, in any form or by any means, without the prior permission of the publisher.

© Copyright by Deutscher Ärzte-Verlag GmbH, Köln 1992

Produced by Deutscher Ärzte-Verlag GmbH, Köln

Contents

Foreword 7

Chapter 1
Explanatory notes on the recordings of findings
(General, oral hygiene, dental fluorosis, trauma to anterior teeth, DMF-T and DMF-S)

1.1	General data sheet	10
1.2	Personal data	12
1.3	Oral hygiene	12
1.4	Dental fluorosis	12
1.5	Trauma to anterior teeth	16

Chapter 2
Tooth data recording

2.1	Data recording sheet "Maxilla"	20
2.2	Data recording sheet "Mandible"	21
2.3	Data on the entire tooth	22
2.4	Data on crown restorations	22
2.5	Data on tooth surfaces	23

Chapter 3
Methods of determining oral health
– Dental caries (on tooth crown)
– The DMF index (DMF-T and DMF-S)

3.1	Carious tooth surfaces (the D component of the index) ...	26
3.2	Missing teeth (the M component of the index)	27
3.3	Filled tooth surfaces (the F component of the index)	27
3.4	Guidelines for data recording	27
3.5	Recording of deciduous teeth	30
3.6	Recording the presence of fissure sealants	30
3.7	Recording procedure – General Rules	31
3.8	Photographs illustrating oral health status recording methods	31

Chapter 4
Removable and non-removable dentures

4.1	Data recording sheet dentures	46
4.2	Entries	47

Chapter 5
Orthodontia

5.1	Data recording sheet orthodontics	50
5.2	Taking impressions of maxilla and mandible	51
5.3	Making entries in the clinical data sheet	52

Chapter 6
Periodontology

6.1	Data recording sheet periodontology	64
6.2	Results of gingival examination (PBI – Papillary Bleeding Index)	65
6.3	CPITN (Community Periodontal Index of Treatment Needs)	65
6.4	Determination of loss of attachment	69
6.5	Illustrations for the explanatory notes under "periodontology" and examples for clinical scoring	73

APPENDIX
Sociological Survey Instruments
for the Assessment of Oral Health Behaviour

– Questionnaire on Oral Health Care and Oral Health Behaviour	80
List of Authors	115

Foreword

The Institut der Deutschen Zahnärzte (Institute of German Dentists – IDZ), Cologne, laid the foundations for the research project "Representative population survey of oral health status and oral hygiene practice in the Federal Republic of Germany" in 1987/88. One of the prerequisites for the implementation of this project was the development of specific instruments, comprising in particular:

a) a Manual detailing the methods of examination and recording of dental data in the fields of cariology, periodontology orthodontics and prosthodontics, and

b) a questionnaire covering the relevant behavioural and sociological aspects.

On completion of the surveys and evaluation of the findings, both the questionnaire and the instructions for examination and data recording proved to have been very effective. As a result of this positive outcome, it was decided to publish the instruments developed for the project in the present volume so as to make them available to interested groups. The Manual has been translated into English, principally because the publishers considered that a Data Recording Manual of this kind might find application in similar projects, including ones conducted in non-German-speaking countries. Another consideration was that comparability with future surveys of oral health status and oral hygiene practice might thus be enhanced.

However, it is hoped that the Manual will also be useful to those concerning themselves with epidemiological questions in the field of oral health for the first time. It will provide them with suggestions and directions that may help them to avoid misconceptions in the planning and conduct of such surveys.

Epidemiological investigations are in any case likely to assume a crucial role within the range of dental research activities in the future. It is, for instance, very important to define the population and age groups that are particularly liable to dental and oral pathology and diseases of the jaw. These risk groups in turn present specific challenges to the social sciences, which are required to analyse the factors deemed responsible, at least in part, for these risk situations.

A detailed mosaic reflecting the oral health or morbidity of the relevant populations, derived from epidemiological surveys, will then constitute a reliable foundation on which subsequent scientific endeavours and health-policy measures can be based.

The Data Recording Manual (Volume 11.2 IDZ-Materialienreihe) is a supplement to the basic scientific publication (Volume 11.1 IDZ-Materialienreihe) describing in detail the methods and the results of the oral health survey conducted by the Institut der Deutschen Zahnärzte in the Federal Republic of Germany in 1989.

Prof. Dr. Rudolf Naujoks, Würzburg

Chapter 1

Explanatory Notes on the Recordings of Findings

(General, oral hygiene, dental fluorosis, trauma to anterior teeth, DMF-T and DMF-S)

1.1 GENERAL DATA SHEET

Institut der Deutschen Zahnärzte

Representative population survey of oral health status and oral hygiene practice in the Federal Republic of Germany

No.: [ ][ ][ ]

Please do not tear out any pages from the Data Book!

Please enter: Subject No.: ☐☐☐ Date of birth: ☐☐ 1 9 ☐☐
                                              Month   Year

Please mark appropriate box with a cross. Like this only: ☒

Sex

Male .... ☐

Female .... ☐

Oral hygiene

1. Good (no plaque visible) .... ☐
2. Poor (plaque clearly visible) .... ☐

Dental fluorosis:

No .... ☐

Uncertain .... ☐

Yes, slight .... ☐

Yes, moderate .... ☐

Yes, severe .... ☐

Trauma to anterior teeth:

Yes .... ☐   No .... ☐
↓
If yes:

Loss of teeth .... ☐   How many teeth?   ◯

Loss of tooth structure ..... ☐   Affecting how many teeth? ◯

No visible damage .... ☐

11

The entries made in the data sheet upon examination are transferred by a scanner to the data storage medium for electronic data processing. It is therefore essential for the entries to be made with *clear* marks.

1.2 Personal data

The following personal data is to be entered in the first data sheet:

a. Subject number
b. Date of birth
    In recording the date of birth, the months from January to September should be represented by 01 to 09.
c. Sex
    For the question: male/female
    please put a cross (x) in the relevant box.

1.3 Oral hygiene

Only two groups are to be formed under this heading. For subject coding, the information for the assistant entering the data should be, for example, as follows:

Upper box or 1 = good

Lower box or 2 = poor

Mark with a cross (x).

1.4 Dental fluorosis

There are five groups for this item:

No:	No staining indicative of dental fluorosis
Uncertain:	Corresponds to figs. 1 a) and b)
Yes, slight:	Corresponds to fig. 1 c)
Yes, moderate:	Corresponds to fig. 1 d)
Yes, severe:	As shown in figs. 1 e) and f)

The boundaries between the individual groups are, of course, fluid.

The teeth should be carefully blown dry before assessment.

Mark with a cross (x).

Note: Mottling of the enamel, at least where slight, must not be equated with fluorosis and must on no account be confused with traumatogenic, hypoplastic white staining of the enamel. For this reason, the principal criteria for the diagnosis of fluorosis are recalled below:

a. The first signs of fluorine-induced alteration of the enamel are whitish lines which accentuate the perikymata and tend to be distributed uniformly over the labial surface of the enamel. If enamel formation is impaired more severely, these lines become wider and coalesce into irregular areas.

b. All these alterations are bilaterally symmetrical.

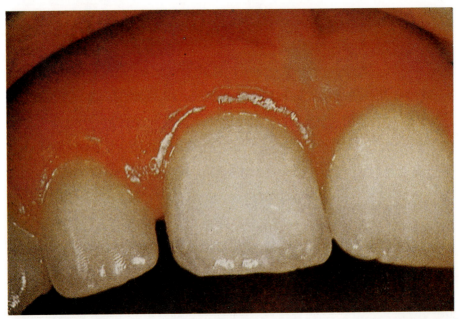

Fig. 1 a–f: Dental fluorosis. The boundaries between the individual degrees of severity are, of course, fluid. The clinical illustrations show examples of the degrees of severity ranging approximately from 0.5 (uncertain) to 4.0 (severe) and correspond to the definitions: uncertain – very mild – mild – moderate – severe.

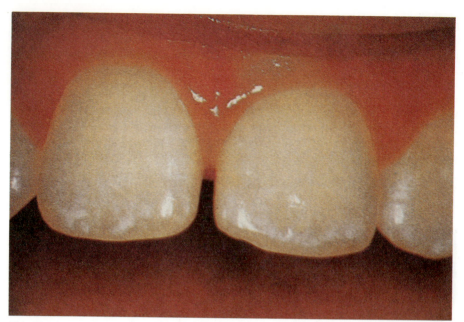

Fig. 1b

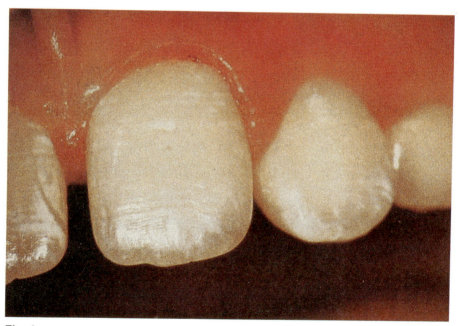

Fig. 1c

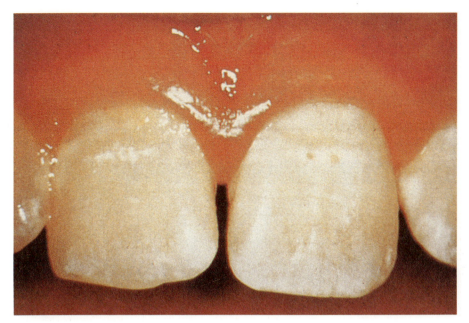

Fig. 1d

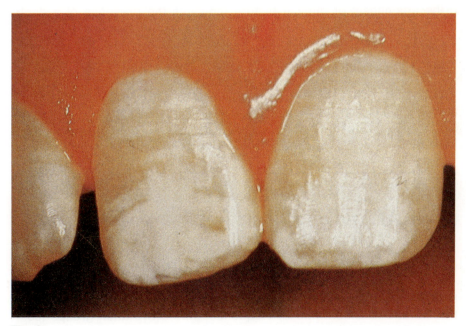

Fig. 1e

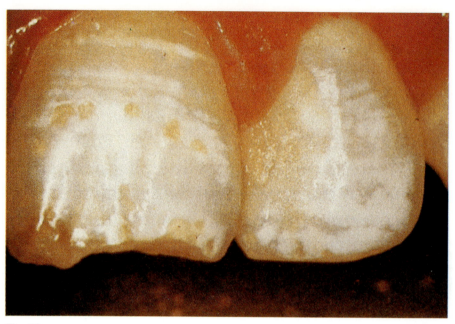

Fig. 1f

1.5 Trauma to anterior teeth

If the anamnesis or clinical picture indicates the presence of a dental trauma, please make the following entries in the relevant boxes (circles):

Trauma to anterior teeth: Yes ☐
                            No ☐

If "yes", please differentiate:

Loss of teeth   ☐   How many teeth?   ◯

Loss of tooth structure   ☐   Affecting how many teeth? ◯
(Crown fracture)

No visible damage   ☐

A cross (x) should be placed in the relevant boxes and the number of teeth affected entered in the circles (example: ②).

N.B. If the anamnesis does not provide clear information as to a dental trauma and its extent and consequences in the two adult groups (35-44 and 45-54 years of age), for instance where the patient already has a complete denture prosthesis or extensive bridgework, please make the following entries:

Trauma to anterior teeth:

Yes ☒ No ☐
If "yes":

↓

Loss of teeth .... ☒ How many teeth? ○
Loss of tooth structure .... ☒ Affecting how many teeth? ○
No visible damage .... ☐

If the information is too vague, simply mark the "no" box under anterior tooth trauma.

Chapter 2

Tooth Data Recording

2.1 Data Recording Sheet "MAXILLA"

2.2 Data Recording Sheet "Mandible"

Each "column" on the data recording sheet represents one tooth. The teeth are identified by the arabic numerals 8-1/1-8.

2.3 Data on the entire tooth

The first field under the tooth identification consists of nine boxes, intended for data on the *entire* tooth.

The abbreviations used for the entries have the following meanings:

F	=	missing tooth (due to caries or for periodontal reasons)
KL	=	extracted for orthodontic reasons or because of trauma, or missing for non-pathological reason
NA	=	congenitally missing tooth
M	=	deciduous tooth
FM	=	deciduous tooth missing, or permanent tooth not yet erupted
Ra	=	retained root
Hy	=	hypoplasia
Er	=	replaced tooth (prosthesis)
Zw	=	pontic

More than one entry may be made for one and the same tooth – e.g., **F** (missing tooth) and **Ra** (retained root).

2.4 Data on crown restorations

The second field under the tooth number, marked "crown" and consisting of four boxes, is intended for information on crown restorations.

The abbreviations used for the entries have the following meanings:

G	=	all-cast or band crown
V	=	veneer crown
J	=	jacket crown (plastics or porcelain)
St	=	post crown

(Mark **G**, **V** or **J**, as appropriate in accordance with the clinical examination, and then, where applicable, add **St** after evaluation of X-rays [if available].)

2.5 Data on tooth surfaces

On the data recording sheet boxes for eight different findings are printed on each tooth surface. More than one item may be marked.

Meaning of abbreviations:

K	=	caries
SK	=	secondary caries
A	=	amalgam filling
G	=	cast filling
Z	=	cement filling
C	=	composite filling
PV	=	temporary filling material
Fi	=	fissure sealant

The surfaces of the teeth should preferably be examined in a particular order.

Suggestion:

Right-hand half of jaw: buccal, *distal*, occlusal, *mesial* and lingual
Left-hand half of jaw: buccal, *distal*, occlusal, *mesial* and lingual

The tooth symbols represent a tooth crown laid out flat.

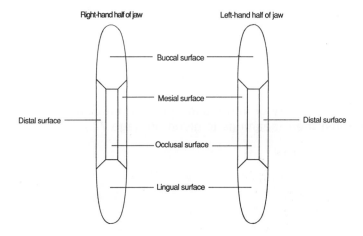

Fig. 2 Tooth Surfaces
There is no occlusal surface in the case of anterior teeth.

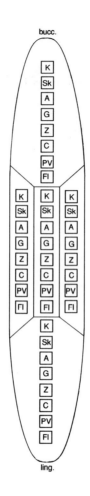

Fig. 3 Coding System

N.B.: In this case all entries should be made with a clear **vertical** mark in the relevant box.

For details, see the next chapter "Methods of determining oral health".

(To facilitate the entry of information in the Data Book, a list of all symbols used and their meanings is given on page 77.)

Chapter 3

Methods of Determining Oral Health

– Dental caries (on tooth crown)
– The DMF index (DMF-T and DMF-S)

The DMF index is an epidemiological instrument for recording data on carious lesions. The DMF-T index is used for entire teeth [T = tooth] and the DMF-S index for tooth surfaces [S = surfaces]. D stands for decayed, M for missing and F for filled.

3.1 Carious tooth surfaces (the D component of the index)

Advanced carious lesions are recognizable as gross cavitations and thus present few problems in diagnosis.

Initial carious lesions, on the other hand, are more difficult to diagnose reliably. These initial stages of caries may be divided into three categories according to location, each with the following diagnostic particularities:

3.1.1 Pits and fissures on occlusal, buccal and lingual tooth surfaces

These areas are diagnosed *as carious when the probe catches after insertion with moderate, uniform pressure and when the catch is accompanied by one (or both) of the following signs of caries:*

a. Softening at the base of the relevant area.
b. Opacity adjacent to the area, indicating undermining or demineralization.

In other words, these pits or fissures in which the probe catches do not in themselves constitute sufficient evidence of caries; they must be accompanied by at least one of the above signs.

3.1.2 Smooth areas on buccal (labial) or lingual surfaces

These areas are deemed carious if a carious defect is visible or identified by careful testing with the probe.

These areas should be deemed sound when there is only visual evidence of demineralization (chalky staining).

3.1.3 Approximal surfaces

For areas accessible to direct visual and tactile examination (e.g., when there is no adjacent tooth), the criteria are the same as those for smooth areas on facial or lingual surfaces.

For areas not available to direct examination, other criteria must be found.

In the case of *anterior teeth*, transillumination can serve as a useful aid in discovering approximal lesions. Transillumination can be achieved by placing the mouth mirror lingually and positioning the examining light so that it passes through the teeth and reflects into the mirror. If a characteristic shadow or loss of translucency is seen on the approximal surface, this is indicative of caries on that surface. If possible, the diagnosis should be confirmed by detection of a defect with the probe. However, the clear shadow of a lesion revealed by transillumination can justify a positive diagnosis.

In *posterior teeth*, however, visual evidence alone, such as undermining under a marginal ridge – is not sufficient proof of the presence of an approximal lesion. A positive diagnosis is possible only if a surface defect can be detected with the probe.

3.2 Missing teeth (the M component of the index)

This component traditionally relates to those permanent teeth that have been extracted only as a result of caries. Because of the difficulty of correctly distinguishing between teeth extracted due to caries and those extracted for periodontal reasons, no attempt should be made to distinguish between these two causes of tooth loss at the time of examination, especially in older subjects. *However, it is essential to distinguish between teeth extracted because of caries or marginal periodontal disease on the one hand and ones extracted for other reasons on the other*. The symbol **F** is used for teeth extracted because of caries or periodontal disease. If teeth are missing because of trauma, orthodontic treatment or other, non-pathological reasons, they are recorded as **KL** ("orthodontic gap"). Congenitally missing teeth are coded **NA** and missing deciduous teeth **FM**.

3.3 Filled tooth surfaces (the F component of the index)

The **F** component represents a tooth surface that has been filled either permanently or temporarily as a result of caries. Here again, it is necessary to distinguish between surfaces restored because of caries and ones filled for other reasons (e.g., trauma, hypoplasia or malformation). Fillings due to trauma, hypoplasia or malformation are *not* recorded.

3.4 Guidelines for data recording

The following conventions have been adopted for the sake of diagnostic consistency:

3.4.1 *Incisal edges of anterior teeth* are not considered to be separate surfaces. If a lesion or filling is confined to the incisal edge, its score should be assigned to the nearest adjacent surface of the relevant tooth. *Anterior teeth* thus have only four scorable surfaces (mesial, distal, labial and lingual). The inclusion of the occlusal surface *of posterior teeth* means that these teeth have five surfaces.

3.4.2 When a carious lesion extends beyond the line angle on to an adjacent surface, this surface is also deemed to be carious. However, an approximal filling on an anterior tooth is not considered to involve the adjacent labial or lingual surface unless at least one third of the crown towards the other approximal surface of the tooth is involved in the filling. The reason for this criterion is that tooth structure on the adjacent surfaces must often be removed to give access for treatment of the approximal lesion on an anterior tooth.

The same applies to approximal surfaces of *posterior teeth*, if access is via the marginal ridge.

To guard against a similar possibility of overscoring in posterior teeth, an approximal-occlusal filling should extend at least a millimetre past the line angle to the adjacent surface before the adjacent buccal or lingual surfaces are also deemed to be involved.

3.4.3 If a permanent tooth has a full crown restoration because of caries, it will be coded **G**, **J**, **V** or **St**. All surfaces of the tooth (four or five depending on the type of tooth) are then counted under the **F** component of the index.

By convention, all *crowns on posterior teeth*, including ones used as bridge abutments or anchors for removable prostheses, are deemed to have been "placed on account of caries". On *anterior teeth*, however, the examiner should investigate why these crowns have been placed. If a crown was placed for any reason other than caries – e.g., fracture, malformation or aesthetics – the reason should not be recorded as caries. If the crown exhibits marginal caries, secondary caries (**SK**) should also be recorded in the relevant position on the data sheet.

3.4.4 *Teeth banded or bracketed* for orthodontic reasons are examined as usual and all visible surfaces scored appropriately.

3.4.5 Certain teeth, especially *first premolars*, are occasionally extracted *in the course of orthodontic treatments*. These teeth are to be *excluded* from the DMF-S analysis. The examiner must make the determination that the teeth were extracted for orthodontic reasons (**KL**). This is not usually difficult owing to the typical symmetry of these extractions.

3.4.6 Non-vital teeth are scored in the same way as vital teeth. However, if a filling on a non-vital tooth was placed solely to seal a root canal and not for caries, this filling should not be scored. If no other lesions or fillings are present, the tooth is deemed sound (caries-free).

3.4.7 Hypoplastic teeth (with defects of form) are recorded as **HY**. However, it may be determined that a filling or crown was placed on such a tooth for *aesthetic reasons* without being necessary because of caries. *In this case the filling/crown is not recorded.*

3.4.8 *Malformed teeth* are recorded in the usual way (e.g., hypoplasia and/or caries). If restored with a full crown for aesthetic reasons, they are *not* recorded.

3.4.9 If a tooth crown has been completely destroyed by caries and *only the root remains, all surfaces are deemed carious.*

3.4.10 If tooth surfaces are both carious and filled, only the caries is scored. If the caries extends from the edge of the filling, score **SK**.

3.4.11 *Fractured or missing fillings* are recorded as if they were intact unless caries is present. In this case the relevant surfaces are deemed to be carious (and not filled).

3.4.12 In the case of *supernumerary teeth*, only one tooth is scored in the relevant position. The examiner must decide which tooth is the "legitimate" occupant of the space.

3.4.13 If both a deciduous and a permanent tooth occupy the same position, *only the permanent tooth is scored.*

3.4.14 *Third molars* are disregarded in determination of the DMF-T index. In examination of first and second molars, it is important to check whether a second or third molar might have drifted mesially, so that it now occupies the position of the first or second molar. In this case, the *first* and *second* molars should be diagnosed and recorded, and not the third. If the second molar has been extracted because of caries and the space is now occupied by the third (sound) molar, the second molar is deemed to have been extracted (code **F**) and the third molar is not recorded.

N.B.: For recording *"tooth restorations"*, the wisdom teeth *are* to be taken into account.

3.4.15 *Stain and pigmentation* alone should not be regarded as symptoms of caries, as they also occur on sound teeth.

3.5 Recording of deciduous teeth

Carious or filled surfaces are recorded in the same way as with permanent teeth, using the same diagnostic criteria. Since many field studies are concerned with both deciduous and permanent teeth, the surface scores for deciduous teeth must be preceded by an **M** (in the headline) to distinguish them from permanent teeth.

The **M** code can then be combined with any other conventional code for caries or filled surfaces.

Example: If a deciduous molar has occlusal caries and is otherwise sound, the **M** code would be combined with the code for occlusal caries. If the deciduous tooth is sound, the **M** code is used alone.

Missing deciduous teeth present problems in recording because it is often not possible to distinguish whether they were lost because of resorption of the roots or caries, especially during the period of mixed dentition. To avoid this problem, deciduous teeth lost up to one year before average physiological exfoliation are recorded as **FM**. For *deciduous teeth lost before this time, both F (missing due to caries) and M (deciduous tooth) are recorded.*

Note again that if *both* a permanent *and* a deciduous tooth are visible in the same space, *only the status of the permanent tooth is recorded*. The deciduous tooth is disregarded.

3.6 Recording the presence of fissure sealants

Fissure seals using adhesive materials should also be recorded. This applies to pits and fissures on posterior teeth and maxillary lateral incisors. The code **Fi** is then recorded in the relevant parts of the data sheet. Sealant on these surfaces is recorded in addition to any other finding. The presence of a sealant should be noted *after* the tooth has been examined for caries.

It is important to realize that different sealant products may vary in appearance (colourless, coloured or white). Sealant should be recorded as present when any part of the surface remains covered. If it appears that *sealant has been used as a filling material* rather than preventively, *the relevant surfaces should be deemed filled* and not *sealed*.

3.7 Recording procedure – General Rules

In the conduct of the examinations, each subject should be examined as far as possible in the same way. For instance, the examiner should resist the temptation to examine a person with severe caries more thoroughly than one who appears less susceptible.

Recommended instruments: A sharp probe, # 23, and a non-magnifying, unscratched mirror. The examination lamp should be positioned to allow transillumination of the approximal surfaces of the anterior teeth from the lingual by means of the mirror. The teeth should be dried in quadrants before examination.

The order of recording should correspond to that of the data sheet. It is a good plan to practise the procedure for overall data recording on a few patients before the main examination commences.

3.8 Photographs illustrating oral health status recording methods

The following photographs illustrate DMF-S assessment (coronal caries). Part of the photos of dental caries were kindly made available to the Institut der Deutschen Zahnärzte by the National Institute of Dental Research, Bethesda, for the purposes of the study (Ref.: National Institutes of Health "Oral Health Surveys of the National Institute of Dental Research: Diagnostic Criteria and Procedures". NIH Publication No. 91-2870, January 1991). We thank the NIDR for the permission to reprint the photos.

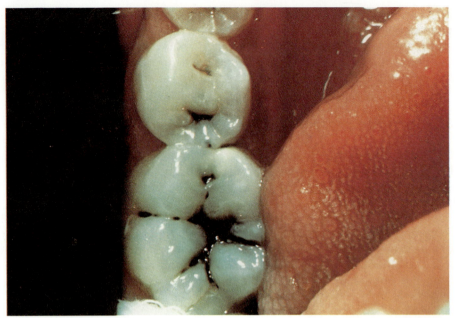

Fig. 4: Caries in the occlusal pits and fissures of the molar and premolar. Each of these teeth would be scored **K** for the occlusal surface. The buccal surface of the molar would receive a **K** if caries is confirmed with the probe. Undermining caries seems to be present on the mesial surface of the first molar, but this must be confirmed with the probe.

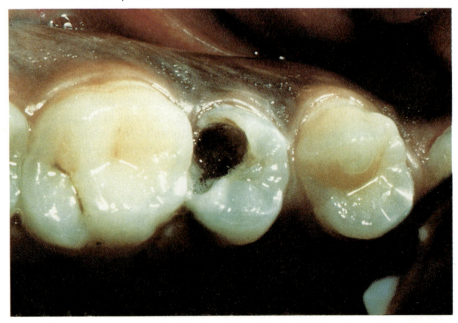

Fig. 5: The second premolar has a large carious lesion extending beyond the line angle on to the buccal surface. This tooth would be scored **K** for the occlusal, buccal and distal surfaces.

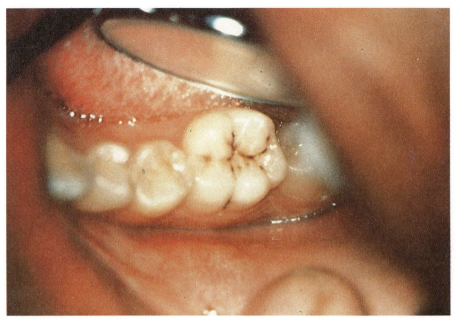

Fig. 6: Stained pits and fissures per se do not constitute a positive diagnosis for caries.

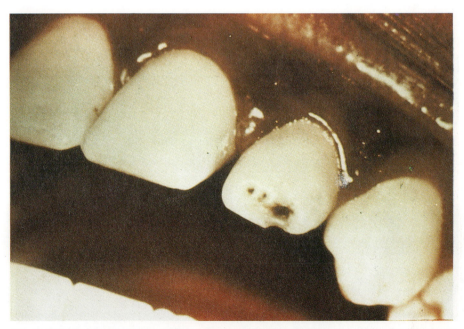

Fig. 7: The lateral incisor has labial caries and hypoplastic pits: code **K** for the labial surface to indicate the location of the lesion.

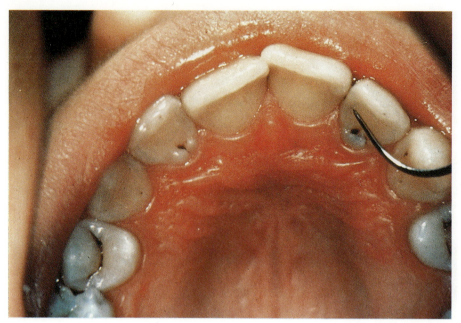

Fig. 8: If the lingual pits in the lateral incisors are found to be carious on exploration with the probe, this surface would receive the code **K**.

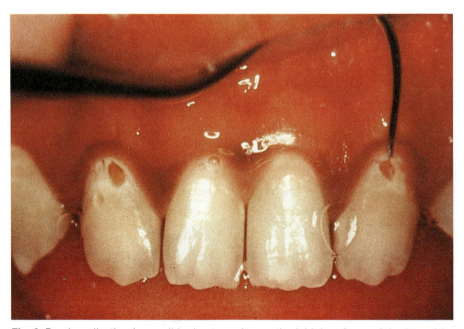

Fig. 9: Demineralization is possibly due to caries on the labial surfaces of the lateral incisors. If a defect is found, the surface is coded **K**.

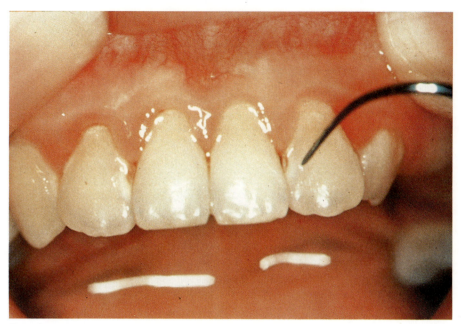

Fig. 10: An approximal lesion on the mesial surface of the lateral incisors would be coded **K**. On anterior teeth, clear visualization of a lesion by transillumination can justify a positive diagnosis.

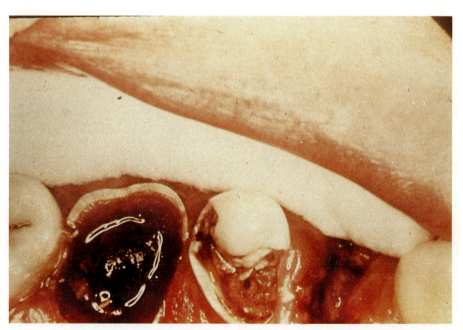

Fig. 11: Only the roots of the first premolar and the first molar are present. Only a part of the crown of the second premolar still exists. In these cases, all surfaces of the relevant teeth would be scored carious.

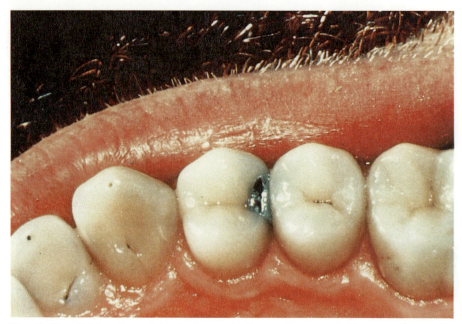

Fig. 12: The distal surface of the first premolar has been restored. The second premolar is caries-free.

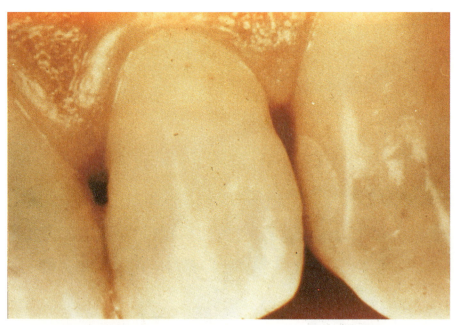

Fig. 13: Composite fillings on the upper lateral incisor and canine. The mesial and distal surfaces of the incisor and the mesial surface of the canine are scored C. The labial surfaces are *not* scored because the filling does not extend one third of the distance across the surface.

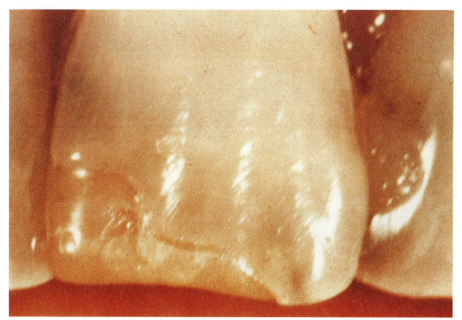

Fig. 14: If the restoration on the central incisor has been placed because of caries, the lingual, labial and mesial surfaces should be marked. (The incisal surfaces are never scored.) If the reason for the restoration was a fracture, it should be ignored and the tooth deemed sound.

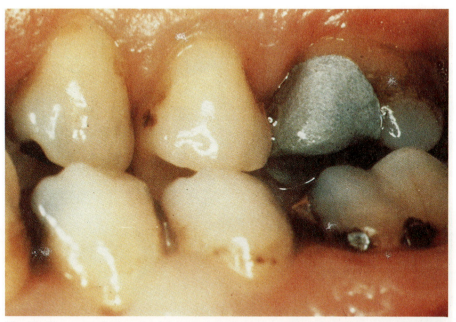

Fig. 15: The upper first molar has a major filling (occlusal, lingual, buccal and mesial). Although two fillings are present on the buccal surface of the lower molar, only one restoration code should be entered, unless there is also caries. In that case the caries takes precedence and **SK** would be recorded.

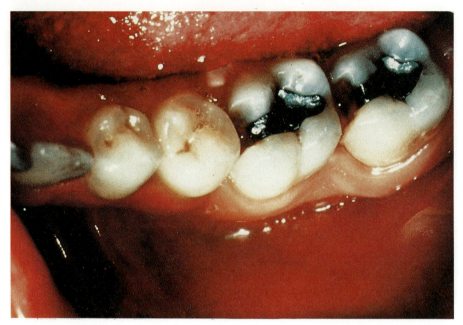

Fig. 16: Fractured amalgam fillings on the first and second molars. If no caries is detected, the teeth should be scored as if the fillings were still intact and present.

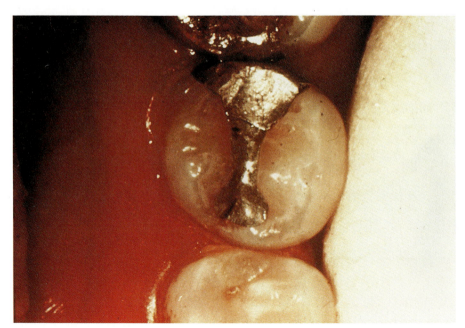

Fig. 17: A distal-occlusal filling with a hairline fracture on a premolar. This tooth is scored as if there were no fracture, unless caries is detected (in which case **SK** would be entered).

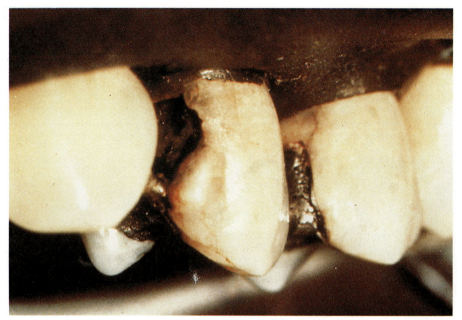

Fig. 18: The mesial surfaces of both premolars have fillings, as well as obvious caries. The caries takes precedence and both surfaces are scored **SK**.

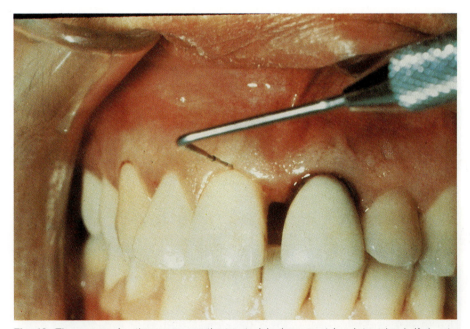

Fig. 19: The reason for the crown on the central incisor must be determined. If due to caries, enter code **V** or **St**. If the crown was placed because of a fracture or for a different, non-disease-related reason, the crown is not recorded.

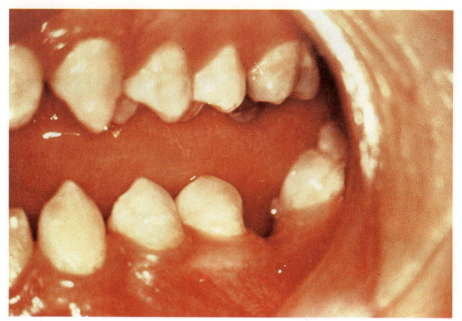

Fig. 20: The lower molar was extracted because of caries and is coded **F**. If it had been extracted for some other reason (non-disease-related), the appropriate entry might be, for example, **KL** (extracted for orthodontic reasons).

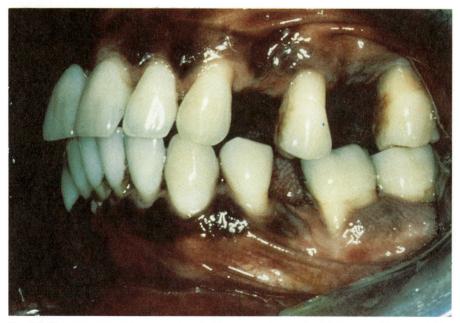

Fig. 21: The missing teeth were extracted because of periodontal disease. They would be scored **F**, as for caries.

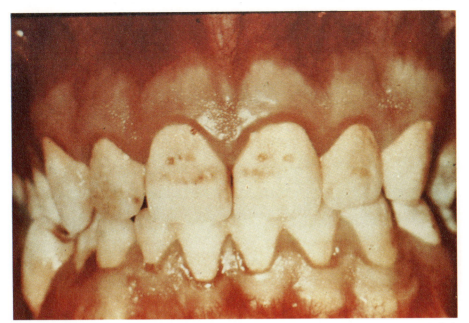

Fig. 22: Hypoplastic teeth are entered as **Hy** unless caries or fillings are present. It is necessary to distinguish whether the filling was placed because of caries or for aesthetic reasons. The filling would be ignored in the latter case.

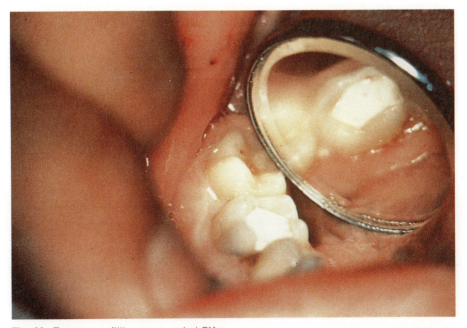

Fig. 23: Temporary fillings are coded **PV**.

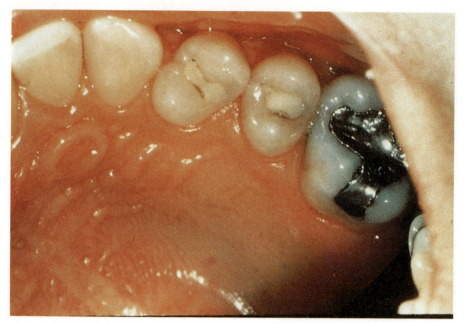

Fig. 24: Composite fillings, or sealants used as filling material, are treated like any other fillings.

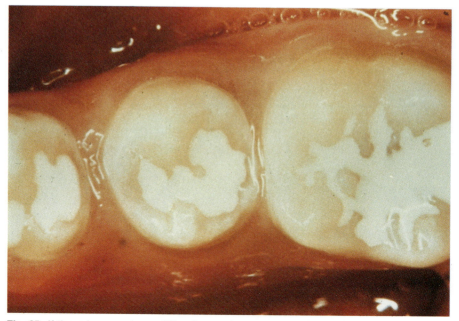

Fig. 25: If there is no caries or filling but sealant material is present, the relevant surface is deemed to have been sealed. This is indicated by the code **Fi**.

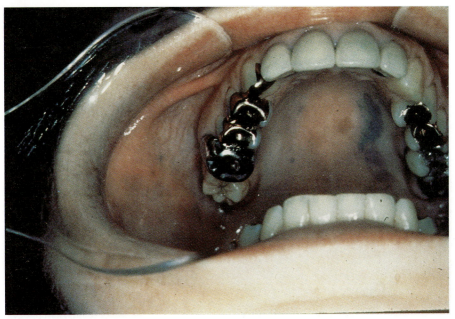

Fig. 26: All full crowns on posterior teeth, including ones with abutments, are coded **G**, **St** or **V**, as appropriate.

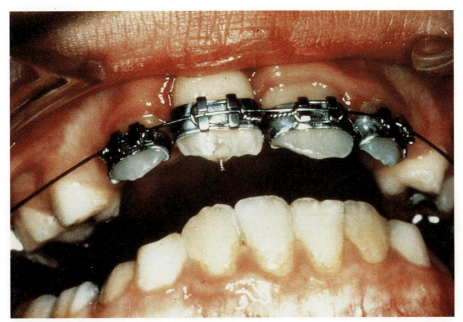

Fig. 27: Orthodontically banded teeth are scored as usual on all visible surfaces. If the upper lateral incisors are deemed to be congenitally missing, they are recorded as **NA**.

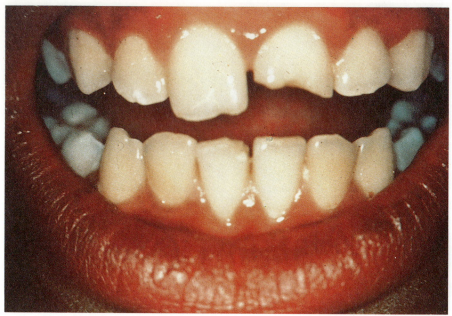

Fig. 28: Untreated fractured teeth are scored as usual on all surfaces. If a full crown has been placed to restore the fracture, the tooth is not recorded. If only the fractured parts of the tooth have been restored, the fillings are ignored and all other surfaces are scored in the usual way.

Chapter 4

Removable and non-removable dentures

4.1 Data Recording Sheet Dentures

Please mark the relevant box with a **cross**. Like this only: [X]

Dentures

Dentures:

Yes .... ☐

No .... ☐ ➡ Please skip this sheet and continue with the chapter "**orthodontia**"

Non-removable dentures:

Zw	Zw	Zw	Zw	Zw	Zw	Zw	Zw		Zw	Zw	Zw	Zw	Zw	Zw	Zw	Zw
K	K	K	K	K	K	K	K		K	K	K	K	K	K	K	K
A	A	A	A	A	A	A	A		A	A	A	A	A	A	A	A
OK 8	7	6	5	4	3	2	1		1	2	3	4	5	6	7	8
UK 8	7	6	5	4	3	2	1		1	2	3	4	5	6	7	8
Zw	Zw	Zw	Zw	Zw	Zw	Zw	Zw		Zw	Zw	Zw	Zw	Zw	Zw	Zw	Zw
K	K	K	K	K	K	K	K		K	K	K	K	K	K	K	K
A	A	A	A	A	A	A	A		A	A	A	A	A	A	A	A

OK = Maxilla
UK = Mandible
Zw = pontic
K = crown (please mark crowns only when they are part of a **bridge construction**, i.e. not single crowns)
A = cantilever

Telescopic bridges:

Yes .... ☐

No .... ☐

Implants:

Yes .... ☐

No .... ☐

Bonded bridges:

Yes .... ☐

No .... ☐

Removable dentures:

Partial

E	E	E	E	E	E	E	E		E	E	E	E	E	E	E	E
OK 8	7	6	5	4	3	2	1		1	2	3	4	5	6	7	8
UK 8	7	6	5	4	3	2	1		1	2	3	4	5	6	7	8
E	E	E	E	E	E	E	E		E	E	E	E	E	E	E	E

OK = Maxilla
UK = Mandible
E = restored tooth

Complete

Maxilla ....   Yes .... ☐   No .... ☐

Mandible ....   Yes .... ☐   No .... ☐

46

4.2 Entries

If the subject has no dentures, all that needs to be entered here is a cross (x), as shown below:

Dentures

   No (x)

In the case of both *non-removable* and *removable* dentures, enter the appropriate codes only for the teeth thereby restored.

N.B. Single crowns do *not* count as dentures.

Crowns with "cantilevers" count as dentures.

"Telescopic bridges", "implants" and "bonded bridges" are intended as additional information.

Please enter telescopic prostheses as "removable dentures".

Distinguish between partial and complete removable dentures.

All entries should be made with a cross (x).

Chapter 5

Orthodontia

5.1 Data Recording Sheet Orthodontics

Please mark the relevant box with a **cross**. Like this only: [X]

Orthodontics:

Occlusal relationship:

	Right		Left	
6	3	3	6	
m	m	m	m	
n	n	n	n	
d	d	d	d	

m = mesial
n = normal
d = distal

	Supporting area, right	Anterior	Supporting area, left
Crowding, maxilla	☐	☐	☐
Crowding, mandible	☐	☐	☐
Tooth spacing, maxilla	☐	☐	☐
Tooth spacing, mandible	☐	☐	☐
Open bite (more than 0.5 mm)	☐	☐	☐
Edge-to-edge bite	☐	☐	☐
Crossbite	☐	☐	☐
"Non-occlusion"	☐	☐	☐
Canines buccally placed, maxilla	☐	☐	☐
Canines buccally placed, mandible	☐	☐	☐
Deep bite	☐	☐	☐
Overjet, 1.5–2 mm	☐	☐	☐
Overjet, up to 5 mm	☐	☐	☐
Overjet, over 5 mm	☐	☐	☐
Midline deviation	☐	☐	☐

The patient is
- satisfied .... ☐
- not so satisfied .... ☐
- dissatisfied .... ☐

with his tooth alignment

The patient's profile
- shows a harmonious maxillomandibular relationship .... ☐
- suggests prognathic malformation .... ☐
- is indicative of a distal mandibular position .... ☐
- shows the characteristics of an angle class II/2 malocclusion ..... ☐

The orthodontic part of the epidemiological survey consists of two stages:

- Taking of impressions of maxilla and mandible
- Making entries in the clinical data sheet

5.2 Taking impressions of maxilla and mandible

5.2.1 Important instructions for procedure with the patient

Disposable trays are to be used for impression-taking; these are being sent to the dentists participating in the project together with the data recording books and other examination materials. Exact impressions of the following are required: the alveolar processes on the vestibular side of both jaws as far as the fold, the *hard palate and the attachment of the soft palate* in the maxilla, and the anatomy of the mandible as far as the root of the tongue. The impression tray should not be removed from the subject's mouth until the alginate has set completely.

To record the *habitual occlusion* (= CO), please use a double pink wax wafer, which should first be fixed with gentle pressure in the patient's maxilla. The subject is then asked to close his jaws slowly; make sure that the wax is bitten through. In cases where the subject tends to shift the mandible ventrally in this process, it is helpful to guide the mandible carefully with a hand.

In the case of *wearers of removable prostheses*, the impressions should be taken with the prosthesis in position in the mouth. If the patient is completely edentulous, it is not necessary to take impressions of the maxilla and mandible.

5.2.2 Mailing

The impressions taken should be wrapped in *moistened rolls of cotton-wool* and packed in plastic bags; they should if possible be sent on the same day (address stickers are being sent to you with the other survey materials) to:

(Address of a dental laboratory)

Please do not forget to enclose with the plastic bag containing the impressions and wax bites the prepared slip *completed with the patient's data (number, date of birth, date of examination and sex)*. If you have for any reason used your own impression trays, we will, of course, return them to you.

5.3 Making entries in the clinical data sheet

The relevant items in the clinical data sheet should be marked with a cross (x).

5.3.1 Occlusal relations of the canines and the six-year molars

Figure 29 shows not only normal occlusion but also examples of distal and mesial occlusal relationships (from Schulze, *Lehrbuch der Kieferorthopädie*, Vol. 1). The steps illustrated (half premolar width/ whole premolar width) are arbitrary, as a whole spectrum of intermediate stages is possible. Any deviation from normal occlusion must be registered as a distal or mesial occlusal relationship. *The occlusal relationships of canines and molars may be different.*

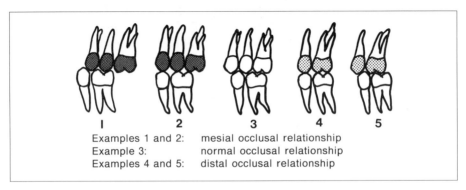

Examples 1 and 2: mesial occlusal relationship
Example 3: normal occlusal relationship
Examples 4 and 5: distal occlusal relationship

Fig. 29: Determination of occlusal relations from Schulze, C: Lehrbuch der Kieferorthopädie, Vol. 1. Quintessenz Berlin, Chicago, Tokyo, 1980

5.3.2 Crowding and spacing in the dental arch

The maxillary *anterior teeth* comprise teeth 11, 21, 12 and 22 and the mandibular anterior teeth are 31, 41, 32 and 42. This means that *the canines are deemed to be posterior teeth*.

Crowding is recorded if a tooth is either outside the row owing to lack of space or does not fit into the row by virtue of its maximum mesiodistal diameter. This is also evident in the case of rotated and tipped teeth which are not in contact with their mesial and distal neighbours (fig. 35).

A tooth is spaced if it does not contact its mesial or distal neighbour in the dental arch.

Where not all teeth are present, crowding and spacing are assessed differently on the basis of development of the dentition for age groups 1

(8-9 years old) and 2 (13-14 years old) on the one hand and 3 (35-44 years old) and 4 (45-54 years old) on the other (figs. 30 and 31).

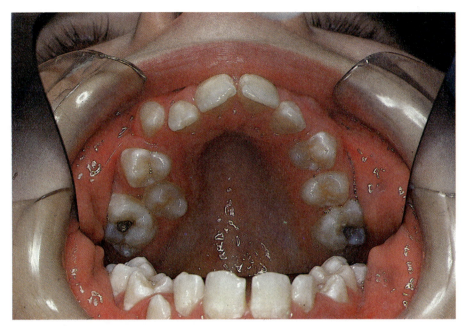

Fig. 30: Crowding and spacing in the dental arch (plan view of maxilla)

Age groups 1 and 2: children and adolescents

In age groups 1 and 2, it is assumed that missing teeth are yet to erupt – that is to say, you must estimate whether there is sufficient room for the permanent teeth or whether the teeth will be crowded or spaced.

Not only crowding that is already visible but also potential secondary crowding due to caries or premature loss of the deciduous molars must be recorded. The relevant clinical criteria are: mesial tipping and rotation of the six-year molars and clearly reduced gaps.

Age groups 3 and 4: adults

In groups 3 and 4, a *prosthetically restored tooth counts as a gap in the same way as a missing tooth*; the gap for the missing tooth may be constricted to a greater or lesser extent.

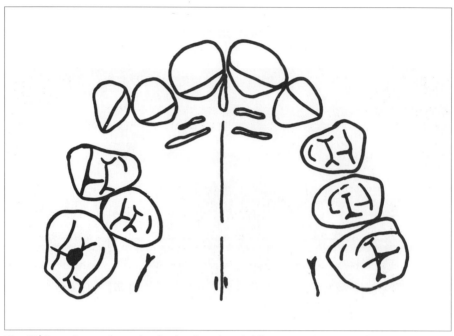

Fig. 31: Crowding and spacing in the dental arch (diagrammatic tracing from fig. 30)

– If the patient belongs to age group 1 or 2 (children and adolescents), you should assume by definition that not all permanent teeth are yet erupted and that tooth 23 is yet to erupt.

The following entries must then be made:

	Supporting area, right	Anterior	Supporting area, left
Crowding, maxilla	X		X
Spacing, maxilla		X	

– If the patient belongs to age group 3 or 4 (adults), you should assume by definition that all permanent teeth have erupted and that the missing tooth 23 is congenitally missing or has been extracted.

The following entries must then be made:

	Supporting area, right	Anterior	Supporting area, left
Crowding, maxilla	X		
Spacing, maxilla		X	X

54

5.3.3 Open bite

If there is no mutual occlusal contact between individual pairs, or several pairs, of antagonists in habitual occlusion – i.e., if there is a vertical gap – the clinical picture of an open bite exists.

This does not apply to teeth in the process of eruption or to deciduous molars which fail to reach the occlusal plane in age groups 1 and 2. If this vertical gap exceeds 0.5 mm in one or more pairs of antagonists, this fact should be recorded in the appropriate column (fig. 32).

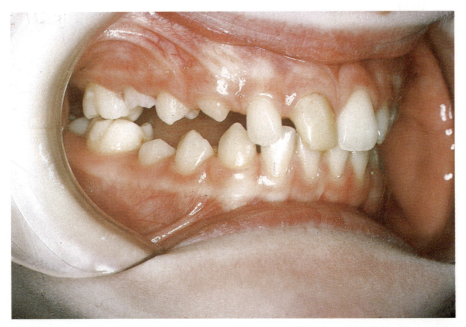

Fig. 32: A clinical picture such as the above is not defined as "open bite" for the purposes of this study, as the premolars and canines are still in the process of eruption and the deciduous molar 55 no longer reaches the occlusal plane.

5.3.4 Edge-to-edge bite/crossbite/"non-occlusion"

These findings relate to transverse deviations of the posterior teeth or sagittal deviations of pairs of anterior antagonists. Fig. 33 illustrates the possible transverse deviations. Examples 1 and 6 would be deemed "non-occlusion", examples 2 and 3 as "crossbite" and example 4 as "edge-to-edge bite".

Example 5 shows the physiological transverse relation of a pair of antagonists. This applies mutatis mutandis to the anterior teeth, except that only "edge-to-edge bite" and "crossbite" are possible in this case.

"Edge-to-edge bite" and "crossbite" are recorded only if there is occlusal contact, while "non-occlusion" is diagnosed without regard to the vertical occlusal relationship (fig. 34).

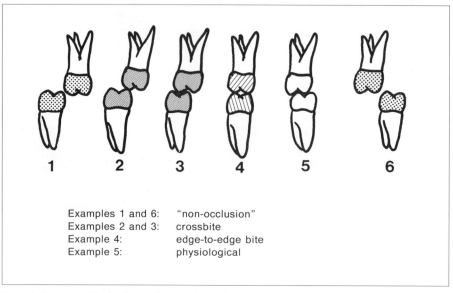

Examples 1 and 6: "non-occlusion"
Examples 2 and 3: crossbite
Example 4: edge-to-edge bite
Example 5: physiological

Fig. 33: Diagram illustrating edge-to-edge bite, crossbite and "non-occlusion" (posterior teeth) from: Schulze, C.: Lehrbuch der Kieferorthopädie. Vol. 1. Quintessenz Berlin, Chicago, Tokyo, 1980

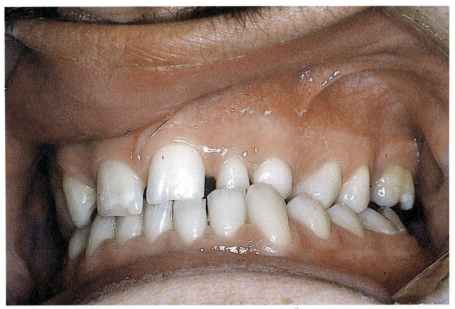

Fig. 34: The canine is deemed to belong to the supporting area by definition. In such a case, a crossbite in the left-hand supporting area must be recorded even if only the canine is in crossbite.

The following entries must then be made:

	Supporting area, right	Anterior	Supporting area, left
Crossbite		X	X

5.3.5 Canines buccally placed

Canines, particularly in the maxilla, may assume a position well outside the overall line of the dental arch owing to the order of eruption (figs. 30 and 35). Once again, only the existence of buccal positioning of the canines is recorded and not its extent.

5.3.6 Deep bite

The overlap of the crowns of the upper and lower incisors is called the overbite. "Deep bite" is entered if, in habitual occlusion, less than half of the subject's mandibular anterior teeth (maxillary anterior teeth in the case of crossbite) is visible (fig. 36).

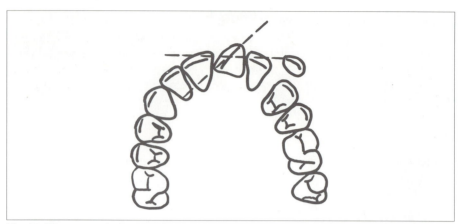

Fig. 35: Diagrammatic tracing of a maxilla with a buccally positioned canine, rotations and crowding; from: Eismann, D: Numerische Erfolgsbewertung kieferorthopädischer Therapie. Med. Habil Dresden, 1978.

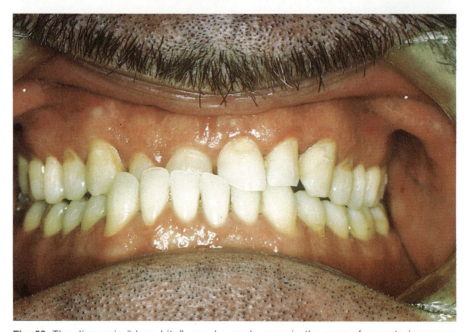

Fig. 36: The diagnosis "deep bite" may be made even in the case of an anterior crossbite. Although the anterior tooth relationship on the left is almost regular, this must be deemed a "deep bite", as the lower anterior teeth mask more than half of their antagonists when viewed from the front.

5.3.7 Overjet

If there is a gap between the crowns of the upper and lower incisors in the sagittal direction in habitual occlusion, this gap is known as a horizontal overbite.

The overjet is measured (1.5 to 2 mm, up to 5 mm or over 5 mm) with a calibrated wooden spatula (calibrated spatulas are being sent to you with the other survey materials), which, resting on the cutting edge of the most labially positioned upper central incisor, is inserted parallel to the occlusal plane until it contacts the labial surface of the antagonist (figs. 37 and 38).

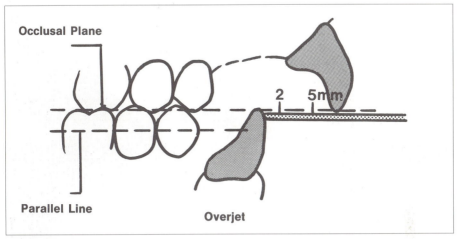

Fig. 37: Diagram illustrating measurement of overjet with the calibrated wooden spatula

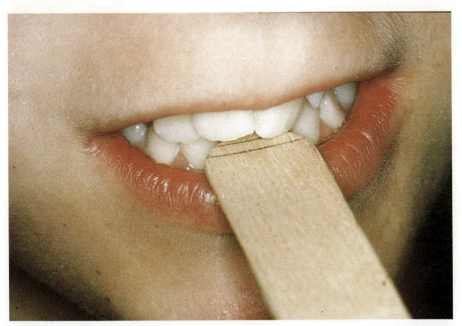

Fig. 38: Procedure for measurement of horizontal overjet with the calibrated wooden spatula (normal overjet)

The same procedure is adopted for frontal crossbite, except that in these cases the spatula is supported on the incisal edges of the lower incisors (fig. 39). The magnitude of the overjet can only be estimated in cases of frontal open bite. Such entries should be preceded with a minus sign ("-x").

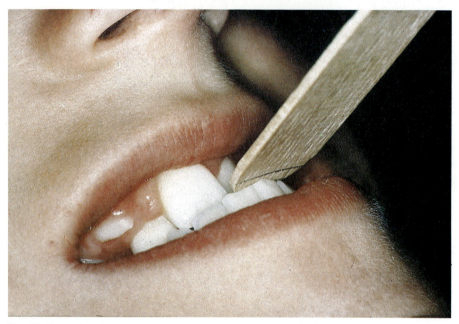

Fig. 39: Procedure for measurement of overjet with the calibrated wooden spatula (anterior crossbite)

5.3.8 Mid lines of maxilla and mandible do not coincide

The mid is always deemed to be the mid line between the upper and lower No. 1 teeth. For this diagnosis, the dentist should view the patient **not from the side but from the front**.

5.3.9 The patient is ..... with his tooth alignment

The subject should be asked whether he is satisfied, not so satisfied or dissatisfied with his tooth alignment, especially that of the anterior teeth (please mark with a cross).

5.3.10 How do you, as the examiner, assess the situation of the patient's profile?

Fig. 40 shows examples of possible profile descriptions. Please disregard the dental findings already arrived at in determining which profile situation is most readily applicable to the subject (please mark with a cross).

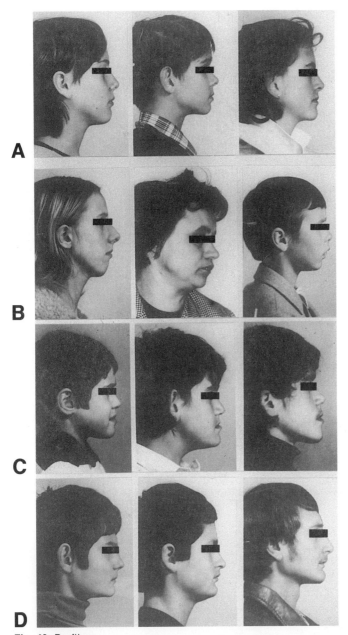

Fig. 40: Profiles:
    A Profile shows a harmonious maxillomandibular relationship
    B Profile slopes backward: Profile suggests distal position of mandible
    C Profile slopes forward: Profile indicative of prognathic malformation
    D Profile shows the characteristics of an angle class II/2 malocclusion

Chapter 6

Periodontology

6.1 Data Recording Sheet Periodontology

Please mark the relevant box with a **cross**.   Like this only: ☒

Periodontology:

Calculus: Yes .... ☐
               No .... ☐

PBI (Papillary Bleeding Index):

F	F	F	F	F	F
0	0	0	0	0	0
1	1	1	1	1	1
2	2	2	2	2	2
3	3	3	3	3	3
4	4	4	4	4	4
OK 16	15	14	13	12	11
UK 46	45	44	43	42	41
0	0	0	0	0	0
1	1	1	1	1	1
2	2	2	2	2	2
3	3	3	3	3	3
4	4	4	4	4	4
F	F	F	F	F	F

OK = Maxilla
UK = Mandible
F = Permanent tooth missing or not yet completely erupted
0 = No blood visible
1 = Single bleeding point, less than 2 mm wide
2 = Two bleeding points or blood on less than half instrumented area
3 = Entire instrumented area full of blood, interdental triangle fills with blood
4 = Severe bleeding upon probing

CPITN (Periodontal Index):

F	F	F
0	0	0
1	1	1
2	2	2
3	3	3
4	4	4
OK 17 16	11	26 27
UK 47 46	31	36 37
0	0	0
1	1	1
2	2	2
3	3	3
4	4	4
F	F	F

F = Permanent tooth (teeth) missing or not yet completely erupted
0 = No bleeding after probing
1 = Bleeding observed either directly or after examination of all sextants
2 = Calculus and overhanging fillings observed during probing; probe cannot be inserted as far as the black area
3 = Pocket depth 4–5 mm; the gingival margin is at the level of the black area of the probe
4 = Pocket depth exceeds 6 mm, black area of probe no longer visible

17	27
47	37
= Please examine these teeth **only in adults**

Only degrees 0, 1 and 2 should be determined in children under 10 years of age.

Attachment (hyperplasia +/recession –):

Teeth	F 17	F 16	F 15	F 14	F 13	F 12	F 11
	B M	B M	B M	B M	B M	B M	B M
+/–							
Rez. (mm)							
TT (mm)							

} Make appropriate **entries** in these boxes; do not put crosses

Rez. = Recession
TT = Pocket depth
F = Permanent tooth missing or not completely erupted

Teeth	F 47	F 46	F 45	F 44	F 43	F 42	F 41
	B M	B M	B M	B M	B M	B M	B M
+/–							
Rez. (mm)							
TT (mm)							

B = buccal
M = mesial

} Make appropriate **entries** in these boxes; do not put crosses

First check whether calculus is present. Put a cross in the appropriate box ("yes" or "no").

6.2 Results of gingival examination (PBI – Papillary Bleeding Index)

Only completely erupted *permanent* teeth should be considered for the examination of children and adolescents. Teeth during eruption are not examined and are coded in the same way as unerupted teeth: **F** (permanent tooth missing or not completely erupted).

Only the first and fourth quadrants are examined. The sulcus is "wiped out" with the tip of the periodontal probe from the buccal aspect of the tooth to the distal aspect of the neighbouring tooth in order to evaluate the papilla. Only slight pressure should be exerted in "wiping" – in magnitude of 20 grams (check the pressure under a fingernail).

Procedure: Retract cheek with the mirror. Dry 16 to 11 from the buccal side with slight air pressure. Start wiping at 16 and continue mesially to 11. Then (after about 10 – 15 seconds) dictate bleeding intensity to assistant. Repeat the same procedure for the mandible (46 to 41).

Recording of results:

F Permanent tooth missing or not yet completely erupted
0 No blood visible
1 Single bleeding point, less than 2 mm wide
2 Two bleeding points or blood on less than half the instrumented area
3 Entire instrumented area full of blood, interdental triangle fills with blood
4 Severe bleeding upon probing

6.3 CPITN (Community Periodontal Index of Treatment Needs)

6.3.1 Indicators

Three indicators of periodontal status are distinguished in examination:

a. Presence or absence of gingival bleeding
b. Supragingival or subgingival calculus
c. Periodontal pockets: divided into medium (4-5 mm) and deep (6 mm or more) pockets.

The examination is carried out with the special-purpose WHO probe (see figure 41).

WHO probe: Lightweight, slender periodontal probe; tip: 0.5 mm diameter sphere, black-painted area between 3.5 mm and 5.5 mm from tip.

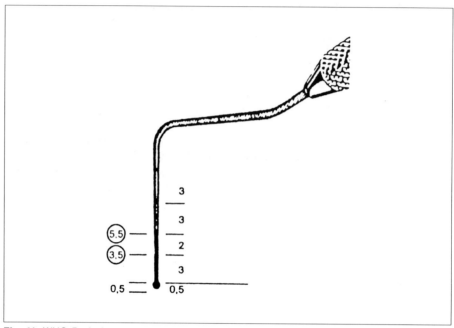

Fig. 41: WHO Periodontal Probe

	F	F	F	F	F	F
	0	0	0	0	0	0
	1	1	1	1	1	1
	2	2	2	2	2	2
	3	3	3	3	3	3
	4	4	4	4	4	4
OK	**16**	**15**	**14**	**13**	**12**	**11**
UK	**46**	**45**	**44**	**43**	**42**	**41**
	0	0	0	0	0	0
	1	1	1	1	1	1
	2	2	2	2	2	2
	3	3	3	3	3	3
	4	4	4	4	4	4
	F	F	F	F	F	F

Fig. 42: Index Teeth (PBI)

6.3.2 Index teeth

Epidemiological surveys do not require examination of all teeth in the sextant, but only index teeth (See figures 42 and 44).

a. Children and adolescents under 20 years of age

The following teeth are examined:

16	11	26
46	31	36

This restriction is intended to avoid the recording of pseudo-pockets as pathological periodontal pockets for example during tooth eruption. For the same reason, pocket depth (degrees 3 and 4) is not determined in children under ten, the examination is restricted to degrees 0, 1 and 2 in these children.

b. Persons over 20 years old

The following teeth are examined:

17	16	11	26	27
47	46	31	36	37

The worst score is recorded in each sextant. If there is no index tooth in the sextant to be examined, all the other teeth in the sextant are examined and the worst CPITN degree is noted. If index teeth are not completely erupted or no other teeth can be examined in the relevant sextant, score **F**. If there are less than two teeth in the sextant the code **F** is also given for the sextant.

6.3.3 Practical procedure

Probing around the index teeth with the WHO probe should be carried out with gentle pressure only (less than 20 grams). A practical test to determine this force is to insert the WHO probe under a thumbnail until the epithelium goes white but no pain is caused. This is an appropriate pressure for probing the pockets or the determination of subgingival calculus. When the WHO probe is inserted (see fig. 43), the sphere must follow the anatomy of the roots. If the patient feels pain, this indicates that too much pressure is being exerted with the probe. There is no rule stipulating at how many aspects a tooth must be probed. This depends

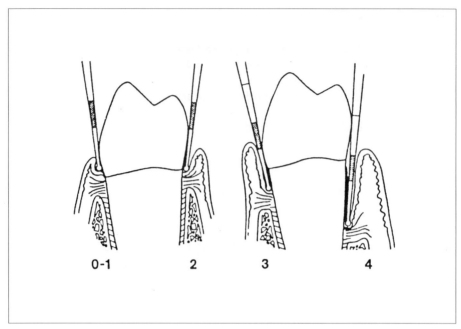

Fig. 43: Exploration of the index teeth with the WHO probe

on the condition of the surrounding gingiva. Sometimes it might be necessary to probe a tooth from all four quadrants.

6.3.4 Examination and recording

The index teeth are examined and the *highest result in each sextant* is recorded:

F Permanent tooth (teeth) missing or not yet completely erupted
0 No bleeding after probing
1 Bleeding observed either directly or after examination of all sextants
2 Calculus and overhanging restorations observed during probing; probe cannot be inserted to the black area
3 Pocket depth 4-5 mm; the gingival margin is at the level of the black area of the probe
4 Pocket depth exceeding 6 mm, black area of probe no longer visible

(on the basis of: Ainamo, J., Barmes, D., Beagrie, G., Cutress, T., Martin, J., Sardo-Infirri, J.: Development of the World Health Organization (WHO) Community Periodontal Index of Treatment Needs (CPITN), Int. Dent. J. 32, 1982, p.281 – 291)

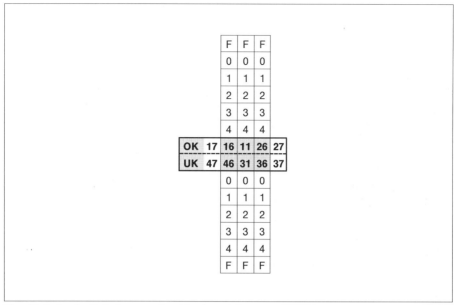

Fig. 44: Index teeth to be examined in the adult group (CPITN)

6.4 Determination of loss of attachment

The determination of loss of attachment is performed at permanent teeth; age group 8-9 years is not examined. Loss of attachment is determined clinically by measuring the distance from the cementoenamel junction to the bottom of the probeable pocket. The loss of connective-tissue attachment is a clinical indication of the destruction of the periodontal tissues. These measurements must be taken from a fixed reference point on the tooth. The most suitable point for this purpose is the cementoenamel junction, as connective-tissue attachment begins here in subjects with healthy periodontal tissues. For the sake of simplicity, the WHO probe can be used again for this purpose. There are marks at 3.5 mm, 5.5 mm, 8.5 mm and 11.5 mm. Measurements are taken in the first and fourth quadrants.

6.4.1 Measuring points

Measurements are taken in the following positions on each tooth:

1. Mesial: The attachment is determined along the axis of the tooth from mesiobuccal. Enter under **M**.

2. The next measurement is carried out on the buccal side of the relevant tooth. Molars should always be measured at the midbuccal aspect of the mesial root. Enter under **B**.

6.4.2 Clinical procedure

First determine whether the gingival margin is above, below or at the cementoenamel junction. Then measure the distance from the cementoenamel junction to the gingival margin. If the gingival margin is below the cementoenamel junction, a *recession* is present and a "−" is entered in the field "+/−". If the gingival margin is above the cementoenamel junction, this indicates *hyperplasia*, in which case a "+" is entered in the field "+/−". If the cementoenamel junction cannot be readily identified, it might be identified by probing up/down with the tip of the WHO probe. If the gingival situation is normal or hyperplasias are present, the tip of the probe (cementoenamel junction) will then be below the margin of the free gingiva. The distance from the cementoenamel junction to the margin of the free gingiva is rounded down to the nearest millimetre and entered in the field **Rez.** (= Recession). If the gingival margin is on the cementoenamel junction, the field "+/−" is left blank and a "0" is entered in the field **Rez.**

6.4.3 Recession

If the gingival margin has receded below the cementoenamel junction, a "−" is entered in the field "+/−". The distance from the gingival margin to the cementoenamel junction is rounded down to the nearest millimetre and entered in the field **Rez.**

6.4.4 Pocket depth

Next the pocket depth is determined. This is done with the CPITN probe along the long axis of the tooth. Enter the measured pocket depth, rounded down to the nearest millimetre, in the field **TT** (Pocket Depth).

6.4.5 Notes

a. Supragingival calculus on the measuring points (**M**; **B**) must be removed before measurement (using a curette).

b. If the cementoenamel junction is concealed by a filling or crown, the examiner should determine its position by comparison with the adjacent teeth or the tooth anatomy and measure the recession or hyperplasia from the resulting reference point.

c. If the cementoenamel junction cannot be determined, the examiner should enter a **F** in the field **Rez.** (Rec.) but still determine the pocket depth.

d. If the natural tooth is missing, enter **F**.

e. Partly erupted teeth and roots retained for reconstructions are not examined (**F**). The cementoenamel junction or a clinical crown must be present at least in part for determination of attachment.

Attachment (hyperplasia +/recession –):

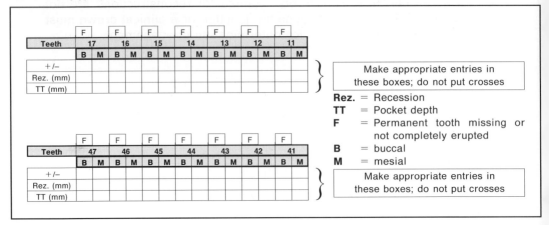

Examples:

	16	15	14	13	12	11
PBI	2	0	3	0	1	0
	4	3	1	1	0	2
	46	45	44	43	42	41

	17/16	11	26/27
CPITN	3	0	1
	3	2	4
	47/46	31	36/37

Attachment (hyperplasia +/recession –):

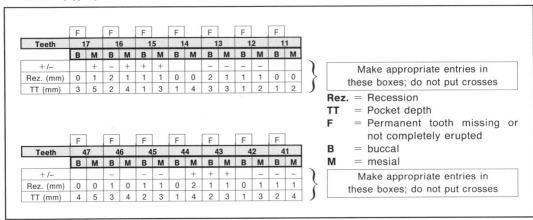

Fig. 45: Examples of entries on the data sheet

6.5 Illustrations for the explanatory notes under "periodontology" and examples for clinical scoring

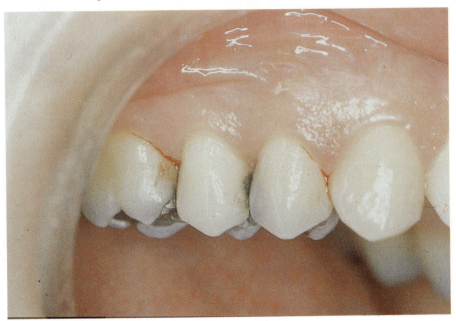

Fig. 46: PBI in Quadrant I
16: Degree 3 / 15: Degree 0 / 14: Degree 2 / 13: Degree 0

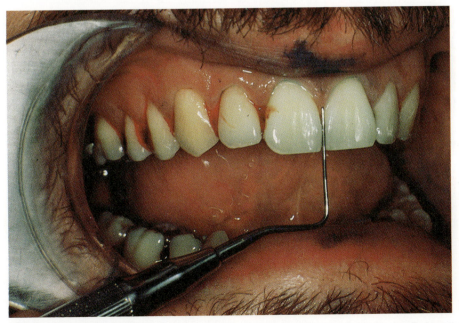

Fig. 47: PBI in Quadrant I
16: Degree 4 / 15: Degree 4 / 14: Degree 2 / 13: Degree 3 / 12: Degree 3 / 11: Degree 2

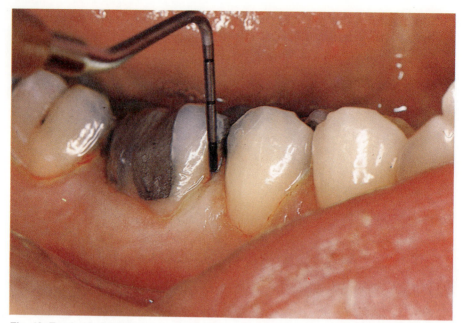

Fig. 48: Tooth 46: CPITN: Degree 1, bleeding after probing pocket less than 3 mm

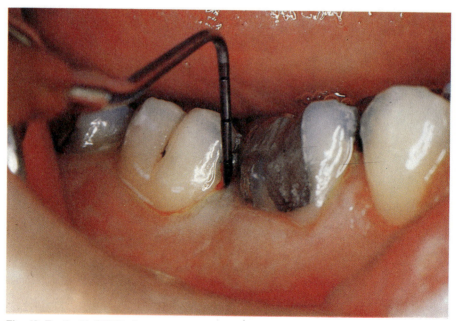

Fig. 49: Tooth 47: CPITN: Degree 3, pocket 4-5 mm

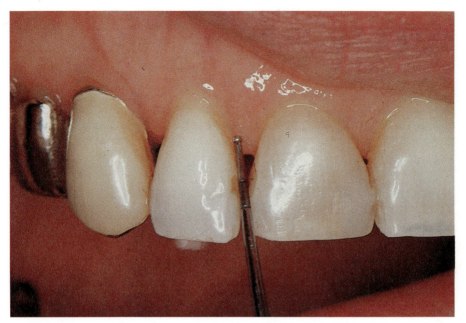

Fig. 50: Attachment: Determination of recession mesial to tooth 12: cementoenamel junction to gingiva: -2 mm

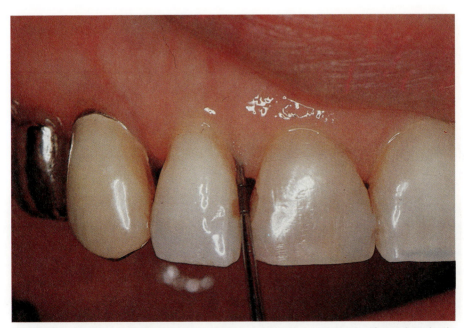

Fig. 51: Attachment: Determination of pocket depth mesial to tooth 12: pocket depth: 2 mm

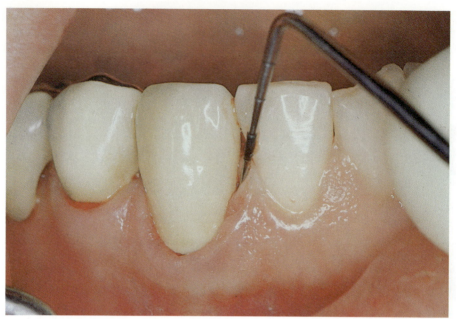

Fig. 52: Attachment: Determination of recession/hyperplasia mesial to tooth 43: if crown margin is subgingivally (approx. 2 mm in the illustration) but the gingiva not hyperplastic (using adjacent tooth for comparison), score ± 0 for recession here.

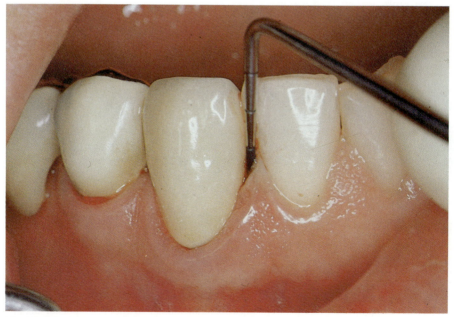

Fig. 53: Attachment: Determination of pocket depth mesial to tooth 43: pocket depth: 4 mm

LIST OF SYMBOLS

F	=	missing tooth (due to caries or for periodontal reasons)
KL	=	extracted for orthodontic reasons or because of trauma, or missing or non-pathological reason
NA	=	congenitally missing tooth
M	=	deciduous tooth
FM	=	deciduous tooth missing, or permanent tooth not yet erupted
Ra	=	retained root
Hy	=	hypoplasia
Er	=	replaced tooth (prosthesis)
Zw	=	pontic
G	=	all-cast or band crown
V	=	veneer crown
J	=	jacket crown (plastics or porcelain)
St	=	post crown
K	=	caries
SK	=	secondary caries
A	=	amalgam filling
G	=	cast filling
Z	=	cement filling
C	=	composite filling
PV	=	temporary filling material
Fi	=	fissure sealant

Appendix

Sociological Survey Instruments for the Assessment of Oral Health Behaviour

Questionnaire on Oral Health Care and Oral Health Behaviour

Authors of the questionnaire:

Dr. Wolfgang Micheelis
Institute of German Dentists, Cologne

Dr. Rosemary Eder-Debye
Infratest Gesundheitsforschung, Munich

Dr. Jost Bauch
Institute of German Dentists, Cologne

The IDZ Oral Health Survey was conducted to determine the prevalences of dental diseases. A particular value of the study is that important attitudes and behavioural aspects in the field of oral health, together with essential sociological factors (e.g.: social stratification!) were also considered. The data were gathered in personal interviews on the basis of a questionnaire (slightly modified according to the different age groups of the study: 8/9 years, 13/14 years, 35 – 44 and 45 – 54 years). For the purposes of the manual publication the basic version, i.e. the questionnaire for the adult group is being reprinted.

Institut der Deutschen Zahnärzte
[Institute of German Dentists]
Universitätsstrasse 71-73
5000 Cologne 41
Telephone 0221/4001(0)

Infratest Forschung
Landsberger Strasse 338
8000 Munich 21
Telephone 089/5600(0)

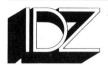

All rights concerning formulation of the questions and the design of the questionnaire are held by **Infratest** and the **Institut der Deutschen Zahnärzte** [Institute of German Dentists]

Project No.: **87/4131/1 February 1989**

Member of the Arbeitskreis Deutscher Marktforschungsinstitute e.V. [Association of German Market Research Institutes]

Please mark as shown: (—)

No.		On to
°0.	The Institut der Deutschen Zahnärzte [Institute of German Dentists] is carrying out a survey of dental health together with Infratest Gesundheitsforschung [Infratest Health Research].°	
°1.	How would you describe your overall state of health? *Please read out possibilities.*° Very good? ( ) Good? ( ) Satisfactory? ( ) Not so good? ( ) Poor? ( )	
°2.	How much is it possible to do oneself to maintain or improve one's **own health**? *Please read out possibilities.*° Very much? ( ) A lot? ( ) A certain amount? ( ) Not much? ( ) Or nothing at all? ( )	
°3.	Thinking particularly of your **teeth**, how would you describe their condition? *Please read out possibilities.*° Very good? ( ) Good? ( ) Satisfactory? ( ) Not so good? ( ) Poor? ( )	

No.		On to

°4.	And how much can one do oneself to maintain or improve the **health of one's teeth**?
	
	| Please read out possibilities.° |
	
	        Very much? ( )
	        A lot? ( )
	        A certain amount? ( )
	        Not much? ( )
	        Or nothing at all? ( )	

°5.	We should now like you to tell us whether you suffer from the following complaints. Please think of **the last four weeks**. Please mark your answers yourself in the following list. | **Present questionnaire to respondent and ask him/her to fill in List 5 him/herself.**°		

Please mark as shown: (—) Please put one mark on **each** line. **List 5**

	Badly	**To some extent**	**Hardly et all**	**Not at all**
Rheumatism	( )	( )	( )	( )
Slipped disc	( )	( )	( )	( )
Stomach trouble	( )	( )	( )	( )
Constipation, sluggishness of bowels	( )	( )	( )	( )
Diarrhoea	( )	( )	( )	( )
Liver or bilious troubles	( )	( )	( )	( )
Kidney troubles	( )	( )	( )	( )
Cystitis	( )	( )	( )	( )
Abdominal troubles	( )	( )	( )	( )
Troubles of the heart and circulation	( )	( )	( )	( )
High blood pressure	( )	( )	( )	( )
Headaches	( )	( )	( )	( )
Toothache	( )	( )	( )	( )
Gum inflammation/gum bleeding	( )	( )	( )	( )
Pain or noises in the jaw joints	( )	( )	( )	( )
Gum shrinkage	( )	( )	( )	( )
Diabetes	( )	( )	( )	( )
Skin problems	( )	( )	( )	( )
Vein problems	( )	( )	( )	( )
Influenza	( )	( )	( )	( )
Cough	( )	( )	( )	( )
Bronchitis	( )	( )	( )	( )
Sore throat, tonsillitis	( )	( )	( )	( )
Head cold	( )	( )	( )	( )
Nausea	( )	( )	( )	( )
Sensitivity to changes in the weather	( )	( )	( )	( )
Disturbances of sleep	( )	( )	( )	( )
Anxiety and nervous tension	( )	( )	( )	( )
States of exhaustion or fatigue, lassitude	( )	( )	( )	( )
Overweight	( )	( )	( )	( )
Underweight	( )	( )	( )	( )

No.					On to
°6.	I shall now read out some habits to you. Please tell me if you do the following ● often ● sometimes ● or never: *Please read out possibilities.*°				
		Often	Some- times	Never	
	Pressing tongue against teeth, cheek, etc.	( )	( )	( )	
	Cheek or lip biting	( )	( )	( )	
	Fingernail biting	( )	( )	( )	
	Pencil chewing	( )	( )	( )	
	Chewing gum	( )	( )	( )	
	Tooth clenching or grinding	( )	( )	( )	
°7.	Are you able to chew any food? Which of the statements in this list applies to you personally? *Present List 7.*° A. Yes, I am able to chew any food ( ) B. No, I have **some** difficulty in chewing ( ) C. No, I have **great** difficulty in chewing ( ) D. Don't know ( )				
°8.	Do you chew mainly – *Please read out possibilities.*° – on both sides? ( )				10
	– on the right? ( )				9
	– or on the left? ( )				
	SPONTANEOUSLY: don't know ( )				10

No.		On to
°9.	If you chew mainly on one side, do you do this because – **Please read out possibilities. More than one answer may be given.°** – teeth are missing? ( ) – teeth are loose? ( ) – the teeth hurt? ( ) – the gums hurt? ( ) – the jaw joint hurts? ( ) – the muscles ache? ( ) – your denture does not stay properly in position? ( ) I don't know why I chew on one side ( )	
°10.	The following list gives some statements. Once again, please mark as applicable to you. **Present questionnaire to respondent and ask him/her to fill in List 10 him/herself.°**	

List 10

Please mark as shown: (—)
Please put one mark on **each** line.

	Happens often	Happens sometimes	Happens rarely	Happens never
When I eat or drink something very hot or very cold, my teeth hurt	( )	( )	( )	( )
My teeth hurt when I clean them	( )	( )	( )	( )
My gums hurt when I clean my teeth	( )	( )	( )	( )
My teeth hurt when I eat sweets	( )	( )	( )	( )

No.		On to
°11.	How far do the following statements apply to you personally now? *Present questionnaire to respondent and ask him/her to fill in List 11 him/herself.°*	

List 11

Please mark as shown: (—)
Please put one mark on **each** line.

	Completely true	Basically true	Partly true	Not really true	Not true at all
I have more trouble with my teeth than other people my age	( )	( )	( )	( )	( )
I think my teeth look good	( )	( )	( )	( )	( )
I am aware that other people notice my tooth alignment/ position	( )	( )	( )	( )	( )
When I am photographed, I try to hide my teeth as far as possible	( )	( )	( )	( )	( )
I do not like my profile very much because of my tooth/ jaw alignment/ position	( )	( )	( )	( )	( )
I have trouble biting off pieces of apple	( )	( )	( )	( )	( )
When eating solid foods (e.g., meat or bread crust), I chew on one side only as a precaution	( )	( )	( )	( )	( )
I cut my meat into as small as possible pieces to make it easier for me to chew	( )	( )	( )	( )	( )

No.		On to
°12.	We should now be interested to hear how often you eat some particular foods. *Present questionnaire to respondent and ask him/her to fill in List 12 him/herself.°*	

Please mark as shown (—)
Please put one mark on **each** line.

List 12

	(Nearly) every day	Several times a week	About once a week	2-3 times a month	Once a month or less	Never
Fish	( )	( )	( )	( )	( )	( )
Meat (except sausage products), poultry	( )	( )	( )	( )	( )	( )
Sausage products, ham	( )	( )	( )	( )	( )	( )
Offals (liver, kidney, heart, brain)	( )	( )	( )	( )	( )	( )
Fresh vegetables (cooked) ..	( )	( )	( )	( )	( )	( )
Deep-frozen vegetables	( )	( )	( )	( )	( )	( )
Canned vegetables	( )	( )	( )	( )	( )	( )
Lettuce, raw vegetables	( )	( )	( )	( )	( )	( )
Fresh fruit	( )	( )	( )	( )	( )	( )
Canned fruit	( )	( )	( )	( )	( )	( )
Coarse-grained wholemeal, black rye, mixed-grain bread (or rolls)	( )	( )	( )	( )	( )	( )
White bread, mixed wheat and rye bread	( )	( )	( )	( )	( )	( )
Oatflakes, muesli (**unsweetened** or with sweetener)	( )	( )	( )	( )	( )	( )
Oatflakes, muesli (sweetened with sugar, honey)	( )	( )	( )	( )	( )	( )
Pasta (noodles, spaetzles) ...	( )	( )	( )	( )	( )	( )
Boiled potatoes (peeled or boiled in their jackets, or mashed)	( )	( )	( )	( )	( )	( )
Fried foods (French fries, croquettes, potato crisps) ...	( )	( )	( )	( )	( )	( )
Rice	( )	( )	( )	( )	( )	( )
Eggs	( )	( )	( )	( )	( )	( )
Cheese	( )	( )	( )	( )	( )	( )
Quark, yoghurt (**unsweetened** or with sweetener)	( )	( )	( )	( )	( )	( )
Quark, yoghurt (**sweetened** with sugar, honey, jam, etc.)	( )	( )	( )	( )	( )	( )
Chocolate	( )	( )	( )	( )	( )	( )
Cake, biscuits, pastry, muesli bars, bread with jam, honey, nougat crème	( )	( )	( )	( )	( )	( )
Ice cream	( )	( )	( )	( )	( )	( )
Blancmange, creamed rice, semolina pudding (**sweetened**)	( )	( )	( )	( )	( )	( )

No.		On to
°13.	And how often do you consume these drinks? *Present questionnaire to respondent and ask him/her to fill in List 13 him/herself.°*	

Please mark as shown (—)
Please put one mark on **each** line.

List 13

	(Nearly) every day	Several times a week	About once a week	2-3 times a month	Once a month or less	Never
Milk	( )	( )	( )	( )	( )	( )
Cocoa drink	( )	( )	( )	( )	( )	( )
Milk shakes, other drinks mixed with milk	( )	( )	( )	( )	( )	( )
Coffee, **sweetened** (sugar)	( )	( )	( )	( )	( )	( )
Coffee, **unsweetened** or with sweetener	( )	( )	( )	( )	( )	( )
Tea, **sweetened** (sugar, honey)	( )	( )	( )	( )	( )	( )
Tea, **unsweetened** or with sweetener	( )	( )	( )	( )	( )	( )
Beer	( )	( )	( )	( )	( )	( )
Wine, Sekt [German sparkling wine], fruit wine	( )	( )	( )	( )	( )	( )
High-strength alcoholic drinks (rum, brandy, liqueur, clear schnaps, etc.)	( )	( )	( )	( )	( )	( )
Fruit juices	( )	( )	( )	( )	( )	( )
Vegetable juices	( )	( )	( )	( )	( )	( )
Mineral water, water	( )	( )	( )	( )	( )	( )
Low-calorie soft drinks (dietetic lemonade, dietetic fruit juice drinks, carbonated drinks with sweetener, cola light, etc.)	( )	( )	( )	( )	( )	( )
Other soft drinks ("ordinary" lemonade, cola, Bluna, Fanta, etc.)	( )	( )	( )	( )	( )	( )

No.		On to
°14.	How often do you eat some kind of snack between meals (breakfast, lunch and evening meal)?	
	Please estimate how many times a day.°	
	Once ( ) Twice ( ) Three times ( ) Four times ( ) Five times or more ( ) Don't know ( )	15
	Don't eat between meals ( )	**16**
°15.	What snacks are your particular favourites?	
	Please read out possibilities.°	
	Bread with sausage or cheese ( )	
	Rolls, pretzels, etc., without filling ( )	
	Fresh fruit or vegetables (raw carrots, etc.) ( )	
	Confectionery (sweets, chocolate, chocolate bars, jelly babies, etc.) ( )	
	Cake, biscuits, waffles, bread with jam, honey, etc., muesli bars ( )	
	Ice cream, blancmange, semolina pudding, creamed rice, etc. ( )	
	Sweetened yoghurt, quark, muesli (with sugar, honey or fruit) ( )	
	Unsweetened yoghurt, quark, muesli, diabetic cakes/biscuits, diabetic chocolate ( )	
	Crisps, flips, peanuts, French fries, etc. ( )	
	Dried fruits, raisins ( )	
	Other **sweetened** snacks ( )	
	Other **unsweetened** snacks (or ones with sweetener) ( )	
	Don't eat between meals ( )	

No.		On to
°16.	What do you particularly like to drink between meals?*	

Please read out possibilities.°

Milk	( )
Cocoa drink	( )
Milk shakes, other drinks mixed with milk	( )
Coffee, **sweetened** (sugar)	( )
Coffee, **unsweetened** or with sweetener	( )
Tea, **sweetened** (sugar, honey)	( )
Tea, **unsweetened** or with sweetener	( )
Beer	( )
Wine, Sekt [German sparkling wine], fruit wine	( )
High-strength alcoholic drinks (rum, brandy, liqueur, clear schnaps, etc.)	( )
Fruit juices	( )
Vegetable juices	( )
Mineral water, water	( )
Low-calorie soft drinks (dietetic lemonade, dietetic fruit juice drinks, carbonated drinks with sweetener, cola light, etc.)	( )
Other soft drinks ("ordinary" lemonade, cola, Bluna, Fanta, etc.)	( )
Other **sweetened** drinks	( )
Other **unsweetened** drinks (or ones with sweetener)	( )
Don't drink between meals	( )

No.								On to
°17.	How often do you chew or suck the following? *Please read out possibilities. Also present List 17.°*							
		A (Nearly) every day	B Several times a week	C About once a week	D 2-3 times a month	E Once a month or less	F Never	
	Chewing gum, with sugar	( )	( )	( )	( )	( )	( )	
	Chewing gum, without sugar	( )	( )	( )	( )	( )	( )	
	Sweets, peppermints, lollipops, etc., **with sugar**	( )	( )	( )	( )	( )	( )	
	Sweets, peppermints, **without sugar**	( )	( )	( )	( )	( )	( )	
°18.	People differ in how often they clean their teeth. What about you? How often do you usually clean your teeth? *Present List 18.°*							
			A 3 times a day or more			( )		
			B Normally twice a day			( )		
			C Normally once a day			( )		19
			D Several times a week			( )		
			E Once a week			( )		
			F Less than once a week			( )		
			G Never (including wearers of full dentures)			( )		26

No.		On to
°19.	When do you usually clean your teeth? **More than one answer may be given.°** After getting up, before breakfast ( ) After breakfast ( ) After lunch ( ) After evening meal ( ) After snacks ( ) Before I go to bed ( ) Varies – when I happen to think of it ( )	
°20.	How long do you clean your teeth for? Please try to estimate the time in minutes or seconds.° About 30 seconds ( ) About 1 minute ( ) About 1½ minutes ( ) About 2 minutes ( ) About 3 minutes ( ) Longer than 3 minutes ( )	
°21A.	Please think about the way you usually clean your teeth. Please try to describe briefly in your own words how you clean your teeth. _____ _____ _____ _____ I always clean my teeth with an electric toothbrush ( )	21B **22**

No.		On to
°21B.	The following list describes some methods of cleaning one's teeth. Please indicate which description most nearly applies to your method. **Present List 21B.** ***More than one answer may be given.**°* A "Scrubbing technique" (wide horizontal to and fro strokes, one stroke extending over a number of teeth or an entire side of the mouth) ( ) B "Shaking technique" (small horizontal to and fro strokes) ( ) C Large, wide circular movements ( ) D Vertical method (vertical movements with the toothbrush held straight) ( ) E Rolling or wiping-out technique – vertical rolling movements "from red to white" (from the gums to the chewing surface) ( ) Other methods I have no fixed system; sometimes I clean my teeth one way and sometimes another ( ) I do not know exactly how I clean my teeth ( )	
°22.	Do you clean your teeth on the outside only or also on the inside?° Outside only ( ) Both sides ( )	
°23.	What about the chewing surfaces? Do you clean the chewing surfaces separately?° Yes ( ) No ( )	

No.		On to

°24A.	For how long do you usually keep your toothbrush?
	
	Where an electric toothbrush is used, the brushhead.
	
	Present List 24A.°
	
	      A 6 weeks or less ( )
	      B 1½ to 3 months ( )
	      C 4 to 6 months ( )
	      D 7 to 12 months ( )
	      E Longer than 12 months ( )	

°24B.	What tells you that you need a new toothbrush?° _____ _____ _____	

°25.	What does your toothbrush look like?
	
	Present illustrations A to E.°
	
	      A . . . . . . ( )
	      B . . . . . . ( )
	      C . . . . . . ( )
	      D . . . . . . ( )
	      E . . . . . . ( )
	      Electric toothbrush ( )
	      Other ( )
	
	A
	B
	C
	D
	E	

No.		On to
°26.	What products do you use for oral hygiene? Please tell me from this list.	

> *Present List 26. More than one answer may be given.*
> *Ask how often only in the case of items D to G.*

Please tell me also how often you use these products.°

                                     I use

A Toothbrush   ( )

B Electric toothbrush   ( )

C Toothpaste, viz:

   ● with fluoride   ( )

   ● without fluoride   ( )

   ● don't know if my
     toothpaste contains fluoride ( )

	I use	Several times a day	(Almost) daily	Several times a week	About once a week	2-3 times a month or less
D Dental floss	( )	( )	( )	( )	( )	( )
E Toothpicks	( )	( )	( )	( )	( )	( )
F Oral irrigator	( )	( )	( )	( )	( )	( )
G Mouthwash	( )	( )	( )	( )	( )	( )
H Other products	( )	( )	( )	( )	( )	( )

No.		On to
°27.	Can you think of anything you can do for your teeth, apart from tooth brushing, to ensure that they stay healthy for as long as possible?° Yes, this: _____ _____ _____ _____ No, I cannot think of anything ( )	
°28.	**Shuffle and present yellow cards.** Some possible ways of preventing oral and dental diseases and troubles are mentioned in these cards. Please try to arrange these possibilities in order of ***importance***. Please put the one that you personally consider most important first, the next most important second, etc. *Form ranking and allow respondent to place all cards in order.*° **Ranking** 1 2 3 4 A Eat no or very little sweets or sugar ( ) ( ) ( ) ( ) B Harden the teeth with fluoride (e.g., fluoride toothpaste, fluoride gel or fluoride tablets) ( ) ( ) ( ) ( ) C Visit dentist for regular check-ups ( ) ( ) ( ) ( ) D Clean teeth properly ( ) ( ) ( ) ( )	

No.		On to
°29.	Have you still got all your natural teeth (other than wisdom teeth)?°	
	Yes ( )	34
	No ( )	30
°30.	**How many** teeth have you **lost** (other than wisdom teeth)? Please include teeth replaced by artificial ones.	
	If respondent cannot give an exact answer, please ask him/her to estimate.°	
	☐☐ Tooth/teeth	
°31.	Do you currently have a fixed or removable dental restoration – i.e., has your dentist fitted you with a crown, bridge or denture?	
	Present List 31. If A is mentioned, please ask, to make sure that the restoration is not removable. More than one answer may be given.°	
	A Fixed denture (cemented in place, e.g. crown, bridge) ( )	
	B Removable denture, viz: • partial denture ( ) • full denture ( )	
	C No denture ( )	

No.				On to
°32.	Have you any gaps in your teeth at present? Please disregard missing wisdom teeth. **N.B.** *Please ask whether a tooth is missing or the teeth are merely widely spaced. Enter "yes" only if teeth are missing.°*			
		Yes	( )	**33**
		No	( )	**34**
°33.	How many of your teeth are missing and have **not** currently been replaced with a restoration (i.e., a crown, bridge or denture)? *If an exact answer is not forthcoming, the respondent should give an estimate.°* ☐☐ Tooth/teeth			
°34.	Has the dentist ever **treated your gums** (treatment for periodontal disease)?°			
		Yes	( )	**35**
		No	( )	**36**
°35.	When was the last time? **Present List 35.°**			
		A I am still being treated	( )	
		B In the last 12 months	( )	
		C In the last 2 years	( )	
		D In the last 5 years	( )	
		E More than 5 years ago	( )	
°36.	Have you ever had any **tooth or jaw regulation or straightening** (i.e., orthodontic treatment)?°			
		Yes	( )	**37**
		No	( )	**41**

No.		On to
°37	Was the treatment carried out with a removable or a fixed appliance or a combination of the two?° With removable appliance ( ) With fixed appliance ( ) With a combination of removable and fixed appliances ( )	
°38.	Have you had permanent teeth removed as part of orthodontic treatment? **Please include wisdom teeth.**° Yes ( ) No ( ) Don't know ( )	
°39.	How long did the treatment take in all? Please tell me from this list. **Present List 39.**° A Less than 1 year ( ) B more than 1 but less than 2 years ( ) C more than 2 but less than 3 years ( ) D more than 3 but less than 4 years ( ) E 4 years or more ( )	
°40.	When did the treatment end? Please tell me again from this list. **Present List 40.**° A I am still in treatment ( ) B In the last 12 months ( ) C In the last 2 years ( ) D In the last 5 years ( ) E More than 5 years ago ( )	
°41.	Has a dentist or dental assistant ever shown you **how** you ought to clean your teeth?° Yes ( )	**42**
	No ( )	**43**

No.		On to

°42.	When was the last time?°
	
	 Present List 42.°
	
	     A In the last 12 months ( )
	     B In the last 2 years ( )
	     C In the last 5 years ( )
	     D More than 5 years ago ( )	

°43.	The next few questions apply to the ordinary dentist and **not** to the orthodontist.
	
	 When did you last go to the dentist?
	
	 Present List 43.°
	
	     A Within the last 12 months ( )
	     B Within the last 2 years ( )
	     C Within the last 5 years ( )
	     D More than 5 years ago ( )
	     E I have never been to the dentist ( )
		44
		
		 47A
		
		 63
		 !

°44.	How often have you been to the dentist in last **12 months**?° [ ] times	

°45.	How often have you been to the dentist in the last **3 months**?°
	
	     [ ] times
	     I have not been to the dentist in the last 3 months ( )
		46
		
		 47A

°46.	How often have you been to the dentist in the last **4 weeks**?°
	
	     [ ] times
	     I have not been to the dentist in the last 4 weeks ( )	

°47A.	Please think of your last visit to the dentist. Was this a single visit or part of a course of treatment?°
	
	     Single visit ( )
	     Course of treatment ( )
	     Can't remember ( )	

No.				On to
°47B.	What was the reason for this visit or course of treatment? **Present List 47B.** **More than one answer may be given.°**	A Acute pain B Repair (e.g., filling dropped out, damage to denture, damage to tooth, etc.) C Scaling D General check-up E Accident/injury F Referral (by doctor) G Other Don't know	( ) ( ) ( ) ( ) ( ) ( ) ( ) ( )	
°48.	What was actually done during your last visit or course of treatment? **Present questionnaire to respondent and ask him/her to fill in List 48 him/herself.**			

List 48

Please mark as follows: (—)
More than one answer may be given

A General examination of teeth .... ( )

B Drilling and filling of one tooth/several teeth .... ( )

C Extraction of one tooth/several teeth .... ( )

D Scaling .... ( )

E Treatment of one or more tooth roots .... ( )

F Gum treatment/treatment for periodontal disease .... ( )

G Tooth or jaw regulation work (orthodontics) .... ( )

H Work for the fitting of *fixed* dentures .... ( )

J Work for the fitting of *removable* dentures .... ( )

K Checking of dentures .... ( )

L Coating of teeth with fluoride varnish .... ( )

M Instruction in mouth and dental hygiene .... ( )

N Other .... ( )

Don't know .... ( )

No.				On to
°49.	Do you go to the dentist only when you have pains or problems, or do you sometimes go for a check-up as well?°			
	I go only when I have pains/problems	( )		51
	I also go sometimes for a check-up	( )		50
	I go for regular check-ups	( )		
	I do not go to the dentist	( )		51
°50.	At what intervals do you go to the dentist for a check-up?			
	Present List 50.°			
	A Every 3 months	( )		
	B Every 6 months	( )		
	C Once a year	( )		
	D Every 2 years	( )		
	E Less often	( )		
	F Irregularly	( )		
°51.	Imagine that you have to go **to the dentist tomorrow**. How do you feel? Please mark the statement that is most applicable to you.			
	Present questionnaire to respondent and ask him/her to fill in List 51 him/herself.°			

List 51

Please mark as shown: (—)

A I quite like going to the dentist .... ( )

B It doesn't bother me .... ( )

C I feel a bit uncomfortable about it .... ( )

D I am afraid it might be painful and unpleasant .... ( )

E I am very anxious and very worried what the dentist might do to me .... ( )

No.		On to
°52.	You have stated that	
	Please refer to Question 51 – for instance, if C was marked: "... that you would feel a bit uncomfortable if you had to go to the dentist tomorrow".	
	Could you explain this in more detail?°	
	_____	
	_____	
	_____	
°53.	Imagine you **are sitting in the dentist's waiting room**.	
	How do you feel? Please mark the statement that is most applicable to you.	
	Present questionnaire to respondent and ask him/her to fill in List 53 him/herself.°	

List 53

Please mark as shown: (—)

A Relaxed .... ( )

B A bit uncomfortable .... ( )

C Tense .... ( )

D Anxious .... ( )

E So anxious that I sweat profusely and feel really ill .... ( )

No.		On to
°54.	Imagine that you are **sitting in the dentist's chair**. The dentist is just preparing the drill to work on your teeth. How do you feel? Please mark the statement most applicable to you. *Present questionnaire to respondent and ask him/her to fill in List 54 him/herself.*°	

List 54

Please mark as shown: (—)

A Relaxed .... ( )

B A bit uncomfortable .... ( )

C Tense .... ( )

D Anxious .... ( )

E So anxious that I sweat profusely and feel really ill .... ( )

No.		On to
°55.	Imagine you are **sitting in the dentist's chair to have scale removed**. While you are waiting, the dentist is getting his instruments ready for scraping off the scale close to the gums. How do you feel? Please mark the statement most applicable to you. *Present questionnaire to respondent and ask him/her to fill in List 55 him/herself.°*	

List 55

Please mark as shown: (—)

A Relaxed .... ( )

B A bit uncomfortable .... ( )

C Tense .... ( )

D Anxious .... ( )

E So anxious that I sweat profusely and feel really ill .... ( )

°56.			
	Please mark according to Lists 51, 53, 54 and 55 (in the questionnaire):°		
	Respondent has mentioned **D** or **E** at least once:		
		Yes ( )	57
		No ( )	**59**

105

No.		On to
°57.	Did you feel that your dentist noticed that you felt anxious or uncomfortable?*	
	Yes ( )	58A
	No ( )	59
	Not sure/don't know ( )	
°58A.	Did the dentist do anything to allay your anxieties?°	
	Yes ( )	58B
	No ( )	59
	Don't know ( )	
°58B.	What did he do?°	
	_____	
	_____	
	_____	
°59.	When you think of your visits to the dentist in the last few years or indeed in earlier years, can you recall anything *particularly unpleasant*? If so, can you give more details and say in what year it was?	
	If an exact time cannot be given, please ask respondent to estimate; even a very rough estimate will do (e.g., "as a child").°	
	Yes, this: _____	
	_____	
	_____ Year _____	
	No, I can't recall anything particularly unpleasant ( )	

No.		On to
°60.	When you think back over your visits to the dentist in the last few years or indeed in earlier years, are there any **pleasant** things which have remained in your memory – for instance, the behaviour of the dentist or of his assistant, the décor of the practice, a particular treatment or treatment result, short waiting times, etc.? If so, can you give details and say in what year? *If an exact date cannot be given, please ask respondent to estimate.°* Yes, this: _____ _____ _____ _____ Year _____ No, can't remember anything pleasant ( )	
°61.	Have you a dentist you would describe as **your** dentist? *Present List 61.°* A I always go to the same dentist for treatment ( )	62
	B I have no permanent dentist, I often change my dentist ( ) C I have no dentist at the moment ( ) D I have never been to the dentist ( )	63
°62.	For how many years have you been going to the same dentist for treatment? *Present List 62.°* A Under 2 years ( ) B 2-4 years ( ) C 5-9 years ( ) D 10-14 years ( ) E 15 years or more ( )	

No.	STATISTICS	On to
°63.	**Sex:**° Male ( ) Female ( )	
°64.	When were you born?° ☐☐ Day ☐☐ Month 19 ☐☐ Year	
°65.	What kind of school-leaving certificate do you have? If you have several, please mention only the **highest**. **Present List 65.**° A Volksschule/Hauptschule [basic school-leaving certificate] ( ) B Mittlere Reife [= approx. "O" level], Realschule [secondary school leaving certificate] ( ) C Entrance qualification for Fachhochschule [specialist college with university status] (leaving certificate of a Fachoberschule [technical school]) ( ) D Abitur [= approx. "A" level] (university entrance) ( ) E Other school-leaving certificate ( ) Not applicable, I have no (or do not yet have a) school-leaving certificate ( )	
°66.	Have you a vocational training qualification or university education? If you have several such qualifications, please mention the **highest**. **Present List 66.**° A Qualification in a trade or in agriculture ( ) B Commercial or other qualification ( ) C Vocational or commercial school qualification ( ) D Qualification of a school in the field of health care ( ) E Technical college (e.g., a training school for master craftsmen or technicians) ( ) F Civil service training qualification ( ) G Fachhochschule [specialist college with university status], school for engineers ( ) H University ( ) J Other education or training qualification ( ) Not applicable; I do not (yet) have a training or educational qualification ( )	

No.	STATISTICS	On to
°67.	Which of the following applies to your present situation?°	
	Present List 67. *More than one answer may be given.*°	
	A Gainfully employed, full-time (all day every working day, even if in family firm – not undergoing training/education) ( )	
	B Gainfully employed, part-time (half-days, a few hours a day, a few days a week, even if in family firm – not undergoing training/education) ( )	
	C Undergoing vocational training (training course/apprenticeship) ( )	
	D In other vocational training (e.g., Fachschule [technical college]) ( )	
	E Registered unemployed ( )	
	F Retired/pensioned off prematurely for health reasons ( )	
	G In voluntary retirement ( )	
	H Housewife (or "househusband") only, not (or no longer) gainfully employed ( )	
	J At school ( )	
	K At university ( )	

No.	STATISTICS	On to
°68.	What is your present job or (if no longer gainfully employed) your last job?	

> Present List 68.°

Worker, non-salaried

A Unskilled worker ( )
B Semiskilled worker ( )
C Skilled and specialized skilled worker ( )
D Foreman ( )
E Foreman with special qualifications, general foreman (civil engineering) ( )

Worker, salaried

F Trained and qualified plant foreman with salaried status ( )
G Salaried worker, basic level (e.g., salesperson, clerk, shorthand typist) ( )
H Salaried worker, higher level (e.g., senior clerk, bookkeeper, technical draughtsman) ( )
J Salaried worker, senior or managerial level (e.g., scientific assistant, officer with statutory powers, head of department) ( )
K Salaried worker with comprehensive management functions (e.g., director, manager, member of the executive board of large undertakings and associations) ( )

Civil servants

L Lower grade ( )
M Clerical grade ( )
N Executive grade ( )
O Administrative grade ( )

Self-employed (including family members helping in family business)

P Self-employed farmers ( )
Q Liberal professions, self-employed academics ( )
R Other self-employed persons with up to 9 employees ( )
S Other self-employed persons with 10 or more employees ( )
T Family members helping in family business ( )

Others (e.g., persons undergoing training and education, schoolchildren, students, persons undergoing military service, persons performing civilian services as a substitute for military service, persons undergoing practical training) ( )

No.	STATISTICS	On to

°69.	What is your marital status?
	
	 Present List 69.°
	
	     A Single, living alone ( )
	     B Single, with permanent partner ( )
	     C Married, living together with spouse ( )
	     D Married, living apart ( )
	     E Divorced ( )
	     F Widowed ( )
		72
		
		 70A

°70A.	What school-leaving certificate does (or did) your partner or spouse have?
	 If he/she has several certificates, please mention only the **highest**.
	
	 Present List 70A.°
	
	   A Volksschule/Hauptschule [basic school-leaving certificate] ( )
	   B Mittlere Reife [= approx. "O" level], Realschule [secondary school leaving certificate] ( )
	   C Entrance qualification for Fachhochschule [specialist college with university status] (leaving certificate of a Fachoberschule [technical school]) ( )
	   D Abitur [= approx. "A" level] (university entrance) ( )
	   E Other school-leaving certificate ( )
	   Not applicable, he/she has no (or does not yet have) a school-leaving certificate ( )	

°70B.	Does or did your partner/spouse have a vocational training qualification or university education?
	 If he/she has several such qualifications, please mention the **highest**.
	
	 Present List 70B.°
	
	   A Qualification in a trade or in agriculture ( )
	   B Commercial or other qualification ( )
	   C Vocational or commercial school qualification ( )
	   D Qualification of a school in the field of health care ( )
	   E Technical college (e.g., a training school for master craftsmen or technicians) ( )
	   F Civil service training qualification ( )
	   G Fachhochschule [specialist college with university status], school for engineers ( )
	   H University ( )
	   J Other education or training qualification ( )
	   Not applicable; he/she does not (yet) have a training or educational qualification ( )	

No.	STATISTICS	On to
°71.	What is the present job of your partner/spouse or (if no longer gainfully employed) what was his/her last job?	

Present List 71.°

Worker, non-salaried

A Unskilled worker ( )
B Semiskilled worker ( )
C Skilled and specialized skilled worker ( )
D Foreman ( )
E Foreman with special qualifications, general foreman (civil engineering) ( )

Worker, salaried

F Trained and qualified plant foreman with salaried status ( )
G Salaried worker, basic level (e.g., salesperson, clerk, shorthand typist) ( )
H Salaried worker, higher level (e.g., senior clerk, bookkeeper, technical draughtsman) ( )
J Salaried worker, senior or managerial level (e.g., scientific assistant, officer with statutory powers, head of department) ( )
K Salaried worker with comprehensive management functions (e.g., director, manager, member of the executive board of large undertakings and associations) ( )

Civil servants

L Lower grade ( )
M Clerical grade ( )
N Executive grade ( )
O Administrative grade ( )

Self-employed (including family members helping in family business)

P Self-employed farmers ( )
Q Liberal professions, self-employed academics ( )
R Other self-employed persons with up to 9 employees ( )
S Other self-employed persons with 10 or more employees ( )
T Family members helping in family business ( )

Others (e.g., persons undergoing training and education, schoolchildren, students, persons undergoing military service, persons performing civilian services as a substitute for military service, persons undergoing practical training) ( )

No.	STATISTICS	On to
°72.	How many persons reside permanently in your household, including yourself? And how many of them are under 18 years old? Please include children.° Total _____ persons of whom _____ persons under 18	
°73.	What is the approximate monthly income of the household – i.e., your net income (all members of the household) after deduction of taxes and social security contributions? **Present List 73.°** A Under 1000 DM ( ) B 1000 to under 1500 DM ( ) C 1500 to under 2000 DM ( ) D 2000 to under 2500 DM ( ) E 2500 to under 3000 DM ( ) F 3000 to under 3500 DM ( ) G 3500 to under 4000 DM ( ) H 4000 to under 4500 DM ( ) J 4500 to under 5000 DM ( ) K 5000 to under 6000 DM ( ) L 6000 DM or more ( ) Refused to answer ( )	
°74.	Are you the main breadwinner?° Yes ( ) No ( )	

No.	STATISTICS	On to
°75.	What kind of health insurance scheme are you insured or included under? Please think also of supplementary insurance schemes and assistance. Mark several items where appropriate. **Present List 75.°** A Local sickness insurance fund (AOK) ( ) B Staff sickness fund ( ) C Guild sickness fund ( ) D Agricultural sickness fund ( ) E Ersatzkrankenkasse [recognized non-State sickness insurance fund] (e.g., Barmer, DAK, etc.) ( ) F Private health insurance scheme ( ) G Assistance ( ) Other (specify): _____ ( ) _____ No sickness insurance ( )	End 76 End
°76.	**For persons with private health insurance only** Are you also insured for dental treatment and dentures (i.e., crowns, bridges and dentures)?° Yes, for dental treatment but not for dentures ( ) Yes, for dental treatment and dentures ( ) No ( ) Don't know ( )	
	[Boxes for statistical notes] _____ ☐☐ ☐☐ 19 ☐☐ Place Day Month Year I confirm that I have conducted the interview correctly and handed the respondent the "Declaration on Data Protection": _____ Interviewer's signature	

List of Authors

Diagnostic Criteria and Data Recording Manual:

Priv.-Doz. Dr. Johannes Einwag
Department of Restorative Dentistry
and Periodontology
University of Würzburg
(Dental caries and dentures)

Dr. Klaus Keß
Department of Orthodontics
University of Würzburg
(Orthodontia)

Dr. Elmar Reich
Department of Restorative Dentistry
and Periodontology
University of Regensburg
(Periodontology)

Sociological Survey Instruments for the Assessment of Oral Health Behavior:

Dr. Jost Bauch, Dipl.-Soz.
Institute of German Dentists
Cologne

Dr. Rosemary Eder-Debye, Dipl.-Psych.
Infratest Gesundheitsforschung
Munich

Dr. Wolfgang Micheelis, Dipl.-Sozw.
Institute of German Dentists
Cologne

Veröffentlichungen des Instituts der Deutschen Zahnärzte

Stand: März 1992

(Die Auflistung schließt die Veröffentlichungen des Forschungsinstituts für die zahnärztliche Versorgung/FZV ein, das seit dem 1. Januar 1987 in das Institut der Deutschen Zahnärzte eingegangen ist.)

Institut der Deutschen Zahnärzte

Materialienreihe

Amalgam – Pro und Contra, Gutachten – Referate – Statements – Diskussion. Wissenschaftliche Bearbeitung und Kommentierung von G. Knolle, IDZ-Materialienreihe Bd. 1, 2. erw. Aufl., ISBN 3-7691-7810-6, Deutscher Ärzte-Verlag, 1988, 1990

Parodontalgesundheit der Hamburger Bevölkerung – Epidemiologische Ergebnisse einer CPITN-Untersuchung. G. Ahrens/J. Bauch/K.-A. Bublitz/I. Neuhaus, IDZ-Materialienreihe Bd. 2, ISBN 3-7691-7812-2, Deutscher Ärzte-Verlag, 1988

Zahnarzt und Praxiscomputer – Ergebnisse einer empirischen Erhebung. S. Becker/F. W. Wilker, unter Mitarbeit von W. Micheelis, IDZ-Materialienreihe Bd. 3, ISBN 3-7691-7813-0, Deutscher Ärzte-Verlag, 1988

Der Zahnarzt im Blickfeld der Ergonomie – Eine Analyse zahnärztlicher Arbeitshaltungen. W. Rohmert/J. Mainzer/P. Zipp, 2. unveränderte Auflage, IDZ-Materialienreihe Bd. 4, ISBN 3-7691-7814-9, Deutscher Ärzte-Verlag, 1988

Möglichkeiten und Auswirkungen der Förderung der Zahnprophylaxe und Zahnerhaltung durch Bonussysteme. M. Schneider, IDZ-Materialienreihe Bd. 5, ISBN 3-7691-7815-7, Deutscher Ärzte-Verlag, 1988

Mundgesundheitsberatung in der Zahnarztpraxis. Th. Schneller/D. Mittermeier/D. Schulte am Hülse/W. Micheelis, IDZ-Materialienreihe Bd. 6, ISBN 3-7691-7817-3, Deutscher Ärzte-Verlag, 1990

Aspekte zahnärztlicher Leistungsbewertung aus arbeitswissenschaftlicher Sicht. M. Essmat/W. Micheelis/G. Rennenberg, IDZ-Materialienreihe Bd. 7, ISBN 3-7691-7819-X, Deutscher Ärzte-Verlag, 1990

Wirtschaftszweig Zahnärztliche Versorgung. E. Helmstädter, IDZ-Materialienreihe Bd. 8, ISBN 3-7691-7821-1, Deutscher Ärzte-Verlag, 1990

Bedarf an Zahnärzten bis zum Jahre 2010. E. Becker/F.-M. Niemann/J. G. Brecht/F. Beske, IDZ-Materialienreihe Bd. 9, ISBN 3-7691-7823-8, Deutscher Ärzte-Verlag, 1990

Der Praxiscomputer als Arbeitsmittel – Prüfsteine und Erfahrungen. M. Hildmann unter Mitarbeit von W. Micheelis, IDZ-Materialienreihe Bd. 10, ISBN 3-7691-7824-6, Deutscher Ärzte-Verlag, 1991

Mundgesundheitszustand und -verhalten in der Bundesrepublik Deutschland – Ergebnisse des nationalen IDZ-Survey 1989. Gesamtbearbeitung: W. Micheelis, J. Bauch. Mit Beiträgen von J. Bauch/ P. Dünninger/R. Eder-Debye/J. Einwag/J. Hoeltz/K. Keß/R. Koch/W. Micheelis/R. Naujoks/K. Pieper/E. Reich/E. Witt, IDZ-Materialienreihe Bd. 11.1, ISBN 3-7691-7825-4, Deutscher Ärzte-Verlag, 1991

Oral Health in Germany: Diagnostic Criteria and Data Recording Manual – Instructions for examination and documentation of oral health status (– with an appendix of the sociological survey instruments for the assessment of oral health attitudes and behaviour –). J. Einwag/K. Keß/E. Reich. IDZ-Materialienreihe Bd. 11.2, ISBN 3-7691-7826-2, Deutscher Ärzte-Verlag, 1992

Psychologische Aspekte bei der zahnprothetischen Versorgung – Eine Untersuchung zum Compliance-Verhalten von Prothesenträgern. Th. Schneller/R. Bauer/W. Micheelis. IDZ-Materialienreihe Bd. 12, 2. unveränderte Aufl., ISBN 3-7691-7829-7, Deutscher Ärzte-Verlag, 1992

Broschürenreihe

Zur medizinischen Bedeutung der zahnärztlichen Therapie mit festsitzendem Zahnersatz (Kronen und Brücken) im Rahmen der Versorgung. Th. Kerschbaum, IDZ Broschürenreihe Bd. 1, ISBN 3-7691-7816-5, Deutscher Ärzte-Verlag, 1988

Zum Stand der EDV-Anwendung in der Zahnarztpraxis – Ergebnisse eines Symposions. IDZ Broschürenreihe Bd. 2, ISBN 3-7691-7818-1, Deutscher Ärzte-Verlag, 1989

Mundgesundheit in der Bundesrepublik Deutschland – Ausgewählte Ergebnisse einer bevölkerungsrepräsentativen Erhebung des Mundgesundheitszustandes und -verhaltens in der Bundesrepublik Deutschland. IDZ Broschürenreihe Bd. 3, ISBN 3-7691-7822-X, Deutscher Ärzte-Verlag, 1990

Sonderpublikationen

Das Dental Vademekum. Hg.: Bundeszahnärztekammer (Bundesverband der Deutschen Zahnärzte)/Kassenzahnärztliche Bundesvereinigung, Redaktion: IDZ, 3. Ausgabe, ISBN 3-7691-4043-5, Deutscher Ärzte-Verlag, 1991

Dringliche Mundgesundheitsprobleme der Bevölkerung in der Bundesrepublik Deutschland – Zahlen, Fakten, Perspektiven. W. Micheelis, P. J. Müller. ISBN 3-924474-00-1, Selbstverlag, 1990*. Überarbeiteter Auszug aus: „Dringlinge Gesundheitsprobleme der Bevölkerung in der Bundesrepublik Deutschland. Zahlen, Fakten, Perspektiven" von Weber, I., Abel, M., Altenhofen, L., Bächer, K., Berghof, B., Bergmann, K., Flatten, G., Klein, D., Micheelis, W. und Müller, P. J. Nomos-Verlagsgesellschaft Baden-Baden, 1990

Dringliche Mundgesundheitsprobleme der Bevölkerung im vereinten Deutschland – Zahlen, Fakten, Perspektiven. A. Borutta/W. Künzel/W. Micheelis/P. J. Müller. ISBN 3-924474-01-X, Selbstverlag, 1991*

Curriculum Individualprophylaxe in der kassenzahnärztlichen Versorgung – eine Handreichung für Referenten zur Fortbildung von Zahnärzten, Zahnmedizinischen Fachhelferinnen (ZMF) und Zahnarzthelferinnen –. J. Einwag/K.-D. Hellwege/J. Margraf-Stiksrud/H. Pantke/H. P. Rosemeier/Th. Schneller, Fachdidaktische Beratung von N. Bartsch, ISBN 3-7691-7827-0, Deutscher Ärzte-Verlag, 1991 (vergriffen)

Forschungsinstitut für die zahnärztliche Versorgung

Materialienreihe

Werkstoffe in der zahnärztlichen Versorgung – 1. Goldalternativen. FZV „Materialien" Bd. 1, ISBN 3-7691-7800-9, Deutscher Ärzte-Verlag, 1980

Eigenverantwortung in der gesetzlichen Krankenversicherung. FZV „Materialien" Bd. 2, Selbstverlag 1980*

Zur Frage der Nebenwirkung bei der Versorgung kariöser Zähne mit Amalgam. FZV „Materialien" Bd. 3, Selbstverlag, 1982 (vergriffen)

Direktbeteiligung im Gesundheitswesen – Steuerungswirkungen des Selbstbehalts bei ambulanten medizinischen Leistungen und beim Zahnarzt. E. Knappe/W. Fritz, FZV „Materialien" Bd. 4, ISBN 3-7691-7803-3, Deutscher Ärzte-Verlag, 1984

100 Jahre Krankenversicherung – Standortbestimmung und Weiterentwicklung des Kassenarztrechts. FZV „Materialien" Bd. 5, ISBN 3-8765-2367-2, Quintessenz Verlag, 1984

Strukturdaten zahnärztlicher Praxen. P. L. Reichertz/K. Walther, FZV „Materialien" Bd. 6, ISBN 3-7691-7807-6, Deutscher Ärzte-Verlag, 1986 (vergriffen)

Broschürenreihe

System der zahnärztlichen Versorgung in der Bundesrepublik Deutschland. B. Tiemann/R. Herber, FZV „Broschüre" 1, ISBN 3-7691-7801-7, Deutscher Ärzte-Verlag, 1980

Kostenexplosion im Gesundheitswesen – Folge eines fehlerhaften Steuerungsmechanismus? J.-M. Graf von der Schulenburg, FZV „Broschüre" 2, ISBN 3-7691-7802-5, Deutscher Ärzte-Verlag, 1981

Merkmale zahnärztlicher Arbeitsbeanspruchung – Ergebnisse einer Fragenbogenstudie. W. Micheelis, FZV „Broschüre" 3, 2. unveränderte Auflage, ISBN 3-7691-7804-1, Deutscher Ärzte-Verlag, 1984

Datenschutz im Gesundheitswesen – Modellversuch zur Erhöhung der Leistungs- und Kostentransparenz. FZV „Broschüre" 4, ISBN 3-7691-7805-X, Deutscher Ärzte-Verlag, 1985

Zukunftsperspektiven der zahnärztlichen Versorgung. FZV „Broschüre" 5, ISBN 3-7691-7811-4, Deutscher Ärzte-Verlag, 1986

Wissenschaftliche Reihe

Medizinische und technologische Aspekte dentaler Alternativlegierungen. C. L. Davidson/H. Weber/H. Gründler/F. Sperner/H. W. Gundlach/P. Dorsch/H. Schwickerath/K. Eichner/G. Forck/R. Kees, FZV „Wissenschaftliche Reihe" Bd. 1, ISBN 3-8765-2366-4, Quintessenz Verlag, 1983

Sonderpublikationen

Übersicht über die Dental-Edelmetallegierungen und Dental-Nichtedelmetallegierungen in der Bundesrepublik Deutschland. Hg. FZV, Deutscher Ärzte-Verlag, 1986 (vergriffen)

*Die Publikationen des Institutes sind im Fachbuchhandel erhältlich. Die mit * gekennzeichneten Bände sind direkt über das IDZ zu beziehen.*